# M.E.N.
## Are the Cause of All Disease

**and other things you don't know about healing**

# DR. SEAN McCAFFREY

Copyright © 2025 Sean McCaffrey

All rights reserved. No part of this publication may be reproduced or transmitted in any form or by any means, electronic or mechanical, including photocopy, recording, or any information storage and retrieval system, without permission in writing from the publisher.

Printed in the United States.

Cover and book design by Asya Blue Design.

ISBN 979-8-9991138-2-5 Hardcover
ISBN 979-8-9991138-1-8 Paperback
ISBN 979-8-9991138-0-1 Ebook

# CONTENTS

FOREWORD . . . . . . . . . . . . . . . . . . . . . . . . . . . . . . . 1

INTRODUCTION: WHO IS DR. SEAN MCCAFFREY? . . . . . . . . . . 11

CHAPTER 1: BLOODLETTING, EPIDEMICS,
              AND THE CHRONIC DISEASES. . . . . . . . . . . . . . . 41

CHAPTER 2: CHRONIC DISEASES
              AND THE EMOTIONS . . . . . . . . . . . . . . . . . . . . . 65

CHAPTER 3: CHOLESTEROL, OPIODS,
              AND THE TRUTH. . . . . . . . . . . . . . . . . . . . . . . . 85

CHAPTER 4: THE OUTLANDISH COST OF
              MEDICAL CARE IN AMERICA . . . . . . . . . . . . . . . 111

CHAPTER 5: THE DIFFERENCE BETWEEN
              ME AND MAINSTREAM MEDICINE . . . . . . . . . . . 135

CHAPTER 6: FROM CONFUSION TO CLARITY:
              AN IUP EXPERIENCE . . . . . . . . . . . . . . . . . . . . . 159

CONCLUSION . . . . . . . . . . . . . . . . . . . . . . . . . . . . . . 189

ABOUT THE AUTHOR . . . . . . . . . . . . . . . . . . . . . . . . . 195

# FOREWORD

*"If you want to find the secrets of the universe, think in terms of energy, frequency and vibration."*

—Nikola Tesla

My name is Dr. Henry Vyner. I am a physician, and I am going to introduce you to one of the most extraordinary healers and physicians I have ever had the pleasure of knowing. His name is Dr. Sean McCaffrey, and he is a man of science and a man of faith. He works with the body, and—because he understands that so much of our body's illness is caused by the workings of the mind—he works with the emotions too.

Dr. McCaffrey has a degree in chiropractic, but he has gone way beyond that degree by studying and mastering several more healing systems he's learned from all over the world. With his doctor bag full of so many different tools, he can heal illnesses that modern medicine has not been able to cure.

There are circles in which some of his methods and theories will be considered unorthodox: He uses acupuncture. He moves energy around in the body. He has diagnostic conversations with a patient's unconscious mind. But what is crucial for us all to focus on and understand is that his methods really work. Consider this example:

Three years ago, Dr. McCaffrey was at a party in Chicago at the home of a friend, Dr. Fox. During the party, Dr. Fox sought out Dr. McCaffrey and asked him to evaluate a good friend of his, a friend who had just recently had surgery to remove a testicular cancer.

Dr. Fox asked Dr. McCaffrey to evaluate his friend Robert because he wanted to know whether Robert had been completely cured—if the cancer had been completely removed—by the surgery. He knew that Dr. McCaffrey would be able to figure out whether Robert was a completely healthy man now.

After some persuasion, Dr. McCaffrey agreed to do an examination right then and there, and at Dr. Fox's insistence, he did it in front of the entire party. Dr. Fox wanted everyone to see just how skilled Dr. McCaffrey is. Fifty people watched as Dr. McCaffrey examined Robert.

Dr. McCaffrey found signs that there were still problems in Robert's body. He found, for example, lymphatic congestion, which in Dr. McCaffrey's medical universe can play a role in causing cancer. He found other problems as well, but he didn't mention any of them out loud to the partygoers who surrounded him as he examined Robert. He didn't want to alarm anyone.

Dr. McCaffrey completed his examination by asking Robert one simple question: "What have you changed in your life since the operation?"

Robert's answer was short and to the point. "Nothing."

Robert was convinced that his surgery had completely cured him, that there was no need to change his nutrition or his daily habits or to take a look at his emotional life in any way. After the surgery, the scans and X-ray reports gave him a clean bill of health, and Robert was doing his utmost to put on a happy face. He exuded a frenetic joy.

The fact that Robert had not examined his life or changed any of his routines or rhythms was a red flag for Dr. McCaffrey, and I'll tell you why in a moment. Dr. McCaffrey told Robert that he would be glad to examine him further if he wished, and that he thought he could help him. Robert thanked him for his offer but told him that he was fine.

"I'm doing awesome!" Robert said. "The surgery worked."

Three months later, Robert showed up at Dr. McCaffrey's door. The tests that his oncologist—his cancer doctor—was doing were showing that the cancer was coming back.

Robert's doctors used two main tests to evaluate whether his cancer was returning: a CT scan and a blood test for a molecule called alpha fetal protein.

The CT scan is used in cancer cases to hunt for metastases. After a surgery to remove the primary site of a cancer, the chance always remains that the cancer is still in your body in some other place. It is the very nature of cancer to hide and to spread, and when it spreads to a new place, it creates what is called a metastasis.

This is what happened to Robert. He had a cancer in one of his testicles. That testicle was the primary site of his cancer, and it was removed by surgery in March 2016. At the time, there were no signs that the cancer had spread. At 9.9, his alpha fetal protein was normal (the normal level for alpha fetal protein is any number below 10), and a CT scan found no metastases.

It's important to remember that cancer can be invisible at first. Here's why: A metastasis is at first just a cluster of a few cells that have broken off from the primary cancer and travelled to another place in the body. Those few cells won't show up on a CT scan because they are, at that early stage, too small to be seen by an X-ray. They will, however, definitely grow in number and eventually show up on an X-ray, as they did in Robert's case.

Just five short months after his surgery, Robert was beginning to show signs that the cancer was returning. His alpha fetal protein was up to 27.

An elevated alpha fetal protein level generally means that you might have a cancer of some kind: a liver cancer, a kidney cancer, a lymphoma, or a testicular cancer. In Robert's case it meant that his testicular cancer was probably returning.

Even scarier, now a mass had shown up in a lymph node in Robert's left groin. That node was just above the testicle that had been removed, and it was in the drainage field of Robert's cancer. If the cancer was going to spread, this was the first place it would go.

At this point, Robert remembered Dr. McCaffrey and decided to go see him. His cancer doctors wanted to start doing chemotherapy and radiotherapy on Robert. He asked them to wait, but he didn't tell them why.

Robert made his first visit to Dr. McCaffrey's office on July 31, 2016, five months after the surgery that removed his testicle. Robert came with his wife, and she continued to accompany him for all his subsequent visits.

Back at the party in Chicago, Dr. McCaffrey had felt certain that the cancer had not finished with Robert. Why? Remember that Robert said he hadn't changed anything in his life at all, which told Dr. McCaffrey there was most likely still a problem. I have heard Dr. McCaffrey say many times that there is almost always an emotional component to cancer. All his mentors had told him so, and in his experience with his own patients that had always held true. In Dr. McCaffrey's words, "If you don't clear the emotions that are stuck in a person's body, you're not going to cure their cancer."

So when Dr. McCaffrey asked Robert, at the party in Chicago, if he had changed anything in his life, what he was really hunting for—what he was hoping to find—was that Robert had searched his soul to see if there were any emotional problems within himself that needed to see the light of day and be resolved. Robert's reply that night assured Dr. McCaffrey there was almost certainly a problem. In fact, he told Robert at the party, "The odds are good that you haven't gotten rid of the stress that caused your cancer in the first place."

We should remember that in the context of modern medicine, it isn't unusual that Robert hadn't looked inward to see if he had any troubling emotions that needed to be dealt with and healed. Most patients—and certainly the great majority of medical doctors—don't believe that emotional stresses can cause cancer. As matters stand today, our state-of-the-art understanding of cancers is that they are caused by mutations—a change in the DNA of a single cell.

Mutations happen all the time in our cells. This is normal. But some of those mutations can cause a normal cell to become a cancer cell, and that's the start of a cancer. One cancer cell divides and becomes two cancer cells. Then two cancer cells divide and become four cancer cells, and it just keeps growing and growing.

Medicine has established that certain kinds of radiation, chemicals, and viruses can cause a mutation that will result in a cancer. However, in general, medicine doesn't see emotional stress as a cause of either mutations or cancer.

Dr. McCaffrey, however, knew from his experience that emotional stress can definitely play a role in creating an environment that allows a cancer to grow. That's why he was virtually certain that Robert's cancer hadn't finished with him, and that Robert was probably going to have a relapse.

As fate would have it, three months later, here was Robert, standing at Dr. McCaffrey's door and asking for help. Dr. McCaffrey went to work on Robert right away, deciding to see Robert twice a week after his office hours, enabling him to see Robert for longer periods of time. In Dr. McCaffrey's words, "He had a life-threatening disease, plus he was driving three hours each way to see me, and I wanted to do my very best for him."

First, before we actually take a look at what Dr. McCaffrey did to treat Robert, I want to show you the timeline of what happened to Robert while he was being treated by Dr. McCaffrey. It will show you, in a straightforward, simple way, whether or not Dr. McCaffrey cured Robert's cancer. I will start the timeline several months before Robert entered into treatment with Dr. McCaffrey:

- March 2016: Robert's right testicle was surgically removed. Before removal, Robert's alpha fetal protein (AFP) was 80, which is astronomically high.
- April 2016: Dr. McCaffrey and Robert met at a house party at Dr. Fox's home.

- July 2016: A follow-up CT scan found a mass in Robert's right groin, and a blood test showed that his AFP was going back up again. It was 27.
    - This was strong proof that a metastasis was growing in Robert's groin and that perhaps there were other, still invisible metastases as well.
    - Robert's oncologist told him that he would like to give him a course of chemotherapy and radiotherapy. Robert asked him to wait.
- July 2016: Dr. Fox called Dr. McCaffrey and told him that Robert would like to see him.
- July 31, 2016: Robert went to Springfield and saw Dr. McCaffrey for the first time; from there on out he began to see Dr. McCaffrey twice a week.
- August 20, 2016: Four weeks after beginning to see Dr. McCaffrey, Robert returned to his cancer doctor to get another CT scan and blood test. The results were mixed.
    - The CT scan showed that the mass in his groin had shrunk to just a dot—a good sign.
    - However, his AFP had skyrocketed and was now 50!
- September 2016: Robert continued treatment with Dr. McCaffrey.
- September 5, 2016: Another CT scan showed that the groin lesion had completely disappeared. Robert's AFP came down but was still above normal.
- October 2016: Robert continued treatment through the entire month with Dr. McCaffrey.
- October 11, 2016: Robert's AFP was dramatically reduced but still elevated.

- October 27, 2016: An ultrasound investigation found that groin mass was definitely gone.
- November 2016: Robert continued treatment through the entire month with Dr. McCaffrey.
- December 2016: Robert continued treatment through the entire month with Dr. McCaffrey.
- December 6, 2016: Another CT scan was done and was normal. Robert's AFP was also normal at 8.0.
  - This was strong evidence that the cancer was no longer present in Robert's body.
- December 22, 2016: Another CT scan and AFP were done and were still entirely normal. Robert's AFP remained normal for the next six months.

This chronology tells us that Dr. McCaffrey received a patient with a history of testicular cancer and emerging signs of recurrence of that cancer in late July 2016. Dr. McCaffrey treated that patient for five months, and during that time all signs of that patient's cancer disappeared. The patient's AFP levels returned to normal, and all signs of any metastasis disappeared from his CT scans. During this period, and afterwards as well, the patient received no treatment for his cancer from his oncologist: no further surgery, no chemotherapy, no radiotherapy.

In January 2017, the patient stopped seeing Dr. McCaffrey. However, Dr. McCaffrey does hear from Robert frequently, and all is well. In the interim, Robert's oncologist concluded that there had been a spontaneous remission of Robert's testicular cancer. In other words, everyone concerned, including Robert's cancer doctors, concluded that the cancer had been cured.

Now, I'm going to start all over again at the beginning and show you almost all the treatments that Dr. McCaffrey gave to Robert during the five months that he saw him. You'll want to hold onto your seat. The treatments that Robert received from Dr. McCaffrey are very different from the treatments he received from his oncologist, or that he would have received from any other oncologist in America or Europe. In Dr. McCaffrey's words, "I didn't go after the cancer."

## THE TREATMENT

Even though Dr. McCaffrey knew that the core of Robert's problem was emotional stress, he worked with Robert on several different levels at once, as he does with all his patients. He treats and balances the whole body.

With Robert, Dr. McCaffrey simultaneously worked on: (1) improving his nutrition; (2) supporting and improving his immune system function; (3) cleaning up his lymphatic system; and (4) finding and clearing the stressors in Robert's emotional life. He also made mechanical adjustments to Robert's spine, adjustments for which chiropractic is well known.

I want to emphasize that Dr. McCaffrey works on several levels at once for a very specific reason. Let me explain why.

To draw a vivid contrast between Dr. McCaffrey and the mainstream cancer doctors who saw Robert, let's remember that the mainstream doctors went right for the cancer. They did laboratory studies and took X-ray images to see if a cancer was present. When they found the cancer, they cut it out. Their entire focus was on finding and removing the cancer.

Dr. McCaffrey's approach to healing a cancer—or any other illness—is very different. Whereas modern medicine focuses on a patient's illness, in this case a cancer, Dr. McCaffrey treats the whole body, and he does so for a very important reason. His whole approach to healing is to help the body heal itself. He sets the body free and empowers it to heal itself by removing the stressors that keep the body from doing what has to be done to heal itself. This is a basic principle of his work. I'll explain.

The human body is well equipped to respond to and heal almost any illness that assaults it. Several systems in the body are designed to do just that. For example, the immune system and the inflammatory response are two related but different systems within the human body that are specifically designed to protect and heal the body. In Dr. McCaffrey's words, "The body has a larger native intelligence that it can use to heal itself."

However, stressors can block the body's natural and native ability to heal itself. In Dr. McCaffrey's universe, three basic types of stress block the body's ability to protect itself from illness: mechanical, emotional, and nutritional stressors. When the body's native intelligence is compromised and blocked by one or more of these stressors, illness will develop in the body.

In Dr. McCaffrey's theory of medicine, this is why we get sick. We get sick when the mechanical, emotional, or nutritional stresses we routinely encounter in life overwhelm the body and block it from healing itself.

Dr. McCaffrey began developing his theory of medicine before he even graduated from high school. Read on as I share how his family life contributed to him becoming the doctor he is today.

—Henry Vyner, MD, MA

# INTRODUCTION

## WHO IS DR. SEAN MCCAFFREY?

**by Dr. Henry Vyner**

*"The doctor of the future will give no medicine, but will interest his patients in the care of the human frame, in diet and in the cause and prevention of disease."*

—Thomas Edison

*"The physician is nature's assistant, not her master."*

—Paracelsus

The education that an American medical student receives is extraordinary. It is a voluminous, empowering body of knowledge that lifts you into the upper levels of the stratosphere and makes it possible for you to save lives. An American medical student consumes oodles and oodles of knowledge—anatomy, physiology, microbiology, pathology, pharmacology, and much more—and consigns it all to memory.

By the time you finish your medical training, a sacred body of knowledge has been entrusted to you, and it gives you that most wonderful of gifts: competence. All of a sudden, after years of working day and night, you have the ability to take care of people. You begin to feel like you can bust through swinging doors into the emergency room and save lives.

It's a wonderful thing to be competent in medicine, to be able to help other human beings. I finished my medical training in the late 1970s, and if you had asked me then, as a new doctor, if medical knowledge would grow and change as much as it has since then, I would have said no.

There are scores of new antibiotics. There are several new imaging techniques. There are new diseases. We know so much more now about the molecular mechanisms of health and disease.

The medicine textbook that I consumed in medical school was a single volume of about 1,400 pages. That same textbook is now two volumes—each of which is more than a thousand pages long.

In other words, medical knowledge has grown exponentially since I finished my training, but ... all that growth has occurred within the same basic model of the body and of medicine. The foundation of medicine today is exactly the same as it was when I was training. It's just that new realms of knowledge have been added to that foundation. More stories were added to the skyscraper.

Dr. McCaffrey's knowledge of medicine and healing grew in a much different way. He started out as a chiropractor, but he has added many different systems of healing to his repertoire as he practiced: nutrition, enzyme therapy, acupuncture, herbal medicine, emotion work, physical medicine, and so much more. He began to see the principles of how healing works.

Dr. McCaffrey kept learning new systems of healing because he was driven by an insatiable quest for knowledge. He wanted to be the best doctor he could possibly be, and he wanted to be able to help *all his patients*.

When Dr. McCaffrey found that he couldn't help one of his patients, he would go out and learn more so that he could help that type of patient in the future. He was remarkably honest with himself about his early failures, and they drove him to keep learning. He is still learning to this very day.

This eternal quest to be a better doctor is, however, just one aspect of the story of Dr. McCaffrey. This is also the story of a young boy who grew up in a boisterous, physical, Irish household. The home in which Dr. McCaffrey grew up was a difficult one that molded him into being a fighter who saw himself as an underdog. His childhood put a chip on his shoulder.

To Dr. McCaffrey's credit, he took those fighting qualities and transformed them. He took the chip that his childhood placed on his shoulder and used it to become a better person, a healer who listens to the "still small voice within" to both diagnose and treat his patients, a doctor who has the ability to heal almost anything that walks through his door. He turned lead into gold. It's an inspiring story.

At the center of the maelstrom in which Dr. McCaffrey grew up was his father, John, an angry, frustrated man who stood an imposing six foot, six inches tall. In contrast, young Dr. McCaffrey was considered quite small for his age. Dr. McCaffrey noted that he often felt his father was "tormented and unsettled," like he was always searching for his path in life but never could quite seem to find it.

John McCaffrey was, in his son's words, "a man with a chip on his shoulder." John's father and mother, although accomplished academics, were strict disciplinarians and rather cold and disconnected emotionally. It's not hard to see why John rebelled against his parents' way of life. In Dr. McCaffrey's words, "He [John] didn't do well with authority.

"I often felt as though my dad, through his own obstinance, never really reached his full potential," Dr. McCaffrey continued, "because he had to do things his own way, and he was forever and always trying to prove that he could." John was a man intent on making sure that you knew he was smarter than you were.

In Dr. McCaffrey's words, his father was "brilliant." John graduated from high school at the age of 15 and tested his way into beginning college as a senior. Although he was obviously bright, John never attended college after his placement exams. He felt that if he could test into his senior year, there was nothing they could really teach him.

This led to a life of moving from job to job and from town to town. John's orneriness made it just about impossible for him to hold onto a job. He had that chip on his shoulder when it came to authority, and he always had to prove he was better. As a result, Dr. McCaffrey's family often found themselves trying to maintain a façade of success while always short on money. They were constantly moving from one place to another, often to "run away from debt" or to start over again and again.

At home, Dr. McCaffrey's father was a strict disciplinarian and often unpredictable. He was moody with high highs and low lows. In Dr. McCaffrey's words, "You were just never really sure which side of my dad you were going to see." At times, John was funny and charming; at other times, he was incredibly and excessively physical and angry. According to Dr. McCaffrey, his dad's anger "more often than not" appeared to be directed toward his mother and himself far more than the rest of the family, making Dr. McCaffrey feel as though he couldn't do much right. As a little boy, Dr. McCaffrey was afraid of his father and didn't know what to do when his dad became unpredictably enraged. Time and time again, Dr. McCaffrey's mother came to his aid. "If it wasn't for my mother, I really don't know how far things may have gone when I was little."

Because of this rough upbringing, Dr. McCaffrey came to see himself as an underdog. He could never win with his father, which made him feel like an underdog in his own home. Dr. McCaffrey felt as though he was always doing something wrong in his father's eyes, and he wasn't allowed to be himself.

All of this put a chip on Dr. McCaffrey's shoulder, passing from one generation to the next. "I got prideful about the spankings. I wasn't going to break. I wasn't going to cry. You can hit me as hard as you want, but even if it hurts me bad, I'm not going to cry."

Dr. McCaffrey's father, through all his own personal torment, was making his son into a boy and then a man who would be just like him: always trying to prove to himself and everyone else that he was as good as any of them. Like many young men brought up by a self-denying disciplinarian, Dr. McCaffrey began to operate on the premise that if he could prove he was better and smarter than everyone else, then he could do things his own way and be himself. For him, this was the way out.

The chip on young Dr. McCaffrey's shoulder was further nurtured by the kids in his neighborhood, growing even larger when they told him stories about the outrageous things his father was doing. His family made it a practice to hide the trouble that John was getting into, so Dr. McCaffrey and his brother had no idea what was really going on until other children teased them about things they knew nothing about. Dr. McCaffrey resented learning about his father's problems from random children trying to bait him, and he fought to defend his father's and family's honor.

Dr. McCaffrey's status as an underdog was cemented in his own mind by one other thing: As a child, he had a stray eye, called a *strabismus* in medical terminology. Mix the uniqueness of his father with a visible physical flaw, and other kids found no lack of ammunition with which to tease and bully him. Dr. McCaffrey continued to fight back. He learned that sometimes he could use his wit and intelligence to gain the upper hand with bullies. At other times, Dr. McCaffrey fought hard, but because he was so small, he mostly lost the physical fights.

Dr. McCaffrey's father threw him into a judo class at the age of nine when all the other students in the class were adults. Dr. McCaffrey says now, "I think he thought I was soft, and that I needed some toughening up."

Dr. McCaffrey took to judo with a passion and quickly became good at it. He liked that he was learning to defend himself, and he would later study—and master—several other forms of the martial arts as well. He has black belts in Okinawan karate, Japanese jujitsu and Chinese kung fu. He has also trained extensively in hapkido, Brazilian jujitsu, Muay Thai, Taekwondo and Kali. More than that, he still practices the arts himself and teaches martial arts to law enforcement agencies, branches of the military, and several other government agencies. Dr. McCaffrey says what he likes best about the martial arts is the chivalry and sense of honor that it instills within its teachers, students, and combatants. I find that telling.

Sean learned more than fighting and honor in those first martial arts classes. They introduced him to the healing arts of Asia. Dr. McCaffrey says that every martial art has a healing side. The indigenous martial arts teachers with whom he studied taught him acupuncture, and they also introduced him to the Asian medical theory that it is the balance of energy within the body that determines whether a person is healthy or sick.

In the early stages, Dr. McCaffrey didn't take the healing side of the martial arts very seriously. He wasn't thinking of himself as a doctor or healer yet, but his experiences of healing in the martial arts did open his mind. They impressed Dr. McCaffrey by showing him just how effective the Asian healing techniques could be. The following story reflects this.

One time, when Dr. McCaffrey was 19, he and a couple other students were doing a kung fu demonstration with kung fu master William Chueng in a small town in Kansas. One of the students was a tiny young lady, and she got kicked in the wrist during a demonstration fight. The wrist immediately swelled up "to the size of a softball."

Dr. McCaffrey describes what happened next: "Chueng asked her to hold out her arm, and he passed his hand back and forth over it several times, and then he said to her, 'Don't worry. You didn't break a bone, and you don't need to go to the hospital and get an X-ray.'" Then Chueng took some herbs out of a duffel bag. He gave them to the girl, told her to heat some vodka when she got back to her hotel room that evening, and put the herbs in the heated vodka. Then, of course, she was to rub the solution onto her wrist, all of which she did. The next morning, the swelling was entirely gone, although the wrist was still a bit stiff.

After one more treatment with the same herbs, the wrist was entirely healed. Dr. McCaffrey says that this experience "captivated me." It left the definite impression upon his young mind that there really was something to the Asian healing arts.

However, Dr. McCaffrey's introduction to the healing arts started long before he began to study the martial arts. His mother came from a family of healers. His maternal grandfather and uncles were all old-school chiropractors. They practiced chiropractic as it was practiced and taught by the founder of the discipline, D.D. Palmer (who his grandfather personally knew), which is much different than the standard-issue chiropractic being practiced nowadays.

More than that, the household of Dr. McCaffrey's youth was steeped in holistic healing. His mother had a bag of medicinal herbs and a little black book of remedies passed down from her mother. Whenever anyone got sick, she hauled out her bag and book of home remedies and medicated them.

His mother also knew a bit of chiropractic and would often do adjustments on young Dr. McCaffrey. If he had a cold, she adjusted him. If he injured an ankle or a knee, she adjusted him. Sometimes his grandfather the chiropractor would come by, and he too would do adjustments on Dr. McCaffrey.

Dr. McCaffrey had a lot of health issues as a child, some of them major. In addition to the strabismus, he also had a tumor on his ankle that had to be surgically removed. His mother and grandfather were constantly taking care of him for one reason or another as his grandfather told him stories about his days as a chiropractor.

For those of you who are not familiar with chiropractic, its bread-and-butter treatment is doing adjustments to the spine. The basic theory of chiropractic is that tiny dislocations of the bones in the spine, called subluxations, cause almost all illness. Period.

The basic idea, in chiropractic theory, is that these subluxations lead to illness within the body by blocking the flow of information that normally moves from the brain to the rest of the body and back to the brain. Chiropractic theory takes the position that this flow of information maintains the body's health, and if that flow of information is blocked or disturbed by subluxations, the body will become unhealthy.

Chiropractors heal their patients by removing these subluxations that cause illness by doing manual adjustments to the spine. We'll have more to say about chiropractic theory and its adjustments later.

Dr. McCaffrey learned how to do adjustments as a youngster, doing his first at the age of 12. Once he learned how to do adjustments, he began doing them to his mother. She, too, had a constant stream of aches and pains.

In other words, Dr. McCaffrey and his mother helped each other through the difficulties that life brought their way, both in the home and the world around them, by healing one another. This made Dr. McCaffrey feel close to his mother, and it also drew him into the practice of healing. This was the beginning of his life as a healer.

Nonetheless, by the time Dr. McCaffrey reached college, it had not yet become clear to him that he was going to become a chiropractor. In fact, he entered college thinking that he was going to become a lawyer, but then he changed his mind and decided to become a medical doctor. To get experience in the field of medicine, he took a summer job at a hospital, but he didn't like what he saw. He felt like medicine wasn't always helping its patients, and he turned away from the idea of becoming a medical doctor.

For a while, he wasn't sure what he was going to do with this life, but then a phone call with his uncle James—who was a chiropractic doctor and a naturopathic physician—set him on his way. He decided to become a chiropractor and enrolled in the College of Chiropractic at Logan University in St. Louis. Now he was beginning to grow into the healing tradition that had been a constant presence in his family.

Unfortunately, at first, Logan turned out to be a disappointment, too. The doctors there weren't what he thought they should be. They didn't practice the old-school chiropractic that he knew from his uncle and his grandfather, who was a real healer in Dr. McCaffrey's eyes. He could treat anything.

The professors at Logan were teaching Dr. McCaffrey and his classmates to confine themselves to the treatment of neck pain, back pain, and headaches—indeed, the niche that chiropractic has come to fill in the landscape of modern health care. Most people do, in fact, go to chiropractors to get relief from back and neck pain.

Dr. McCaffrey, in contrast, grew up in a milieu in which chiropractors took on and treated just about anything, and that was what he himself wanted to do. He wanted to be a real healer. This is why he got disillusioned with chiropractic and Logan; for a while, he thought seriously about quitting.

Once again, his uncle came to the rescue, advising him in yet another important phone call to stay in school and "get your license" so that he could practice. Dr. McCaffrey took his advice and decided to stay at Logan, where he finished his degree. Later, he would end up serving on Logan's Alumni Board of Directors.

At this earlier moment, though, when Dr. McCaffrey was disillusioned with chiropractic as it was being taught to him at Logan, we see the first professional outburst of the traits that he developed in childhood.

Dr. McCaffrey had that chip on his shoulder and was invested in proving to people that he was as good as—if not better than—them. And that is what he was feeling at Logan when he first got there. He thought that there must be more than the pedestrian sort of chiropractor that Logan was training him to be.

I asked Dr. McCaffrey once if he really saw himself as an underdog. His answer was an emphatic YES. He said that, after all, he came from a family that had no standing and that he chose for himself "a profession that's the black sheep of the medical world." By doing so, he was going to have to fight for legitimacy for the rest of his life.

But notice: Even within the black-sheep profession of chiropractic, there was still that chip on his shoulder. Dr. McCaffrey thought he could prove he was so much more than the chiropractic profession into which he was being inducted at Logan.

That chip—that desire to prove his worth, to prove that he was capable of so much more—would, in the end, serve Dr. McCaffrey well. It could have been disruptive. It could have led him to be endlessly contentious and pretentious at Logan. It could have led him to drop out, just as his father dropped out of college before him.

Instead, Dr. McCaffrey harnessed that drive to prove himself and used it to better himself. He took that chip on his shoulder and transformed it into a drive to become the best doctor he could possibly become. That naked ambition to simply establish his superiority was the lead that Dr. McCaffrey slowly but surely transformed into gold. With the passage of time, that ambition became the gold of wisdom, wisdom that would turn Dr. McCaffrey into a truly transcendent healer.

Despite his misgivings, and following his uncle's advice, Dr. McCaffrey went on to become an excellent student at Logan, and chiropractic would become the foundation of his medical practice.

While at Logan, Dr. McCaffrey paid a great deal of attention to doing spinal adjustments, and he became excellent at them. Although there are several different systems of doing adjustments in the world of chiropractic, Logan taught only two of them, but by the time Dr. McCaffrey left Logan, he had found a way to study and become proficient at dozens of others. However, Sean would not stop with learning more than his share of adjustment techniques.

He wanted to be able to do more than adjustments, and ironically enough, his first opportunity to expand beyond the traditional confines of chiropractic came while he was at Logan. He created that first opportunity, and when it arose, he grabbed it with both hands.

In addition to being a school that educates new chiropractors, Logan also offers postdoctoral courses to practicing chiropractic physicians that give these established doctors opportunities to learn more. This includes courses in acupuncture, nutrition, kinesiology, and much more. Courses could last for a weekend, a month, a few months, or even a year or more.

As a student wanting to learn as much as possible, Dr. McCaffrey got permission to take these post-doctoral courses. These courses cost money, but Dr. McCaffrey arranged to pay his tuition by working at them—helping to set up, collect tickets at the door, and so forth.

One of the courses he took was a yearlong one on nutrition. In the midst of the course, the instructor fell ill and was replaced by another chiropractor from Wisconsin. His name was Howard Loomis.

At the beginning of his first lecture, Dr. Loomis said, "Forget everything you know about nutrition. We're going to talk about enzymes, amino acids, and proteins." This was different, and Dr. McCaffrey sat up and took notice.

It turned out that Dr. Loomis' approach to nutrition really was different from the usual fare. According to Dr. McCaffrey, in general, nutrition is taught and practiced in a "cookbook" fashion. If you have a cold, you are told to take vitamin C and echinacea. If you have bronchitis, the recipe is to inhale steam saturated with eucalyptus and coltsfoot. Take ginseng for longevity and energy, and so on.

Dr. Loomis' approach was different. He focused on understanding the biochemistry of digestion as a means of improving a patient's overall health, and he prescribed enzymes, herbals, and whole foods to improve digestion. Dr. Loomis invented what has come to be known as the field of enzyme therapy.

Dr. McCaffrey was drawn to Dr. Loomis. He thought Loomis was "skeptical" like himself, as well as "brilliant." He was particularly taken by the fact that no one could punch holes in Dr. Loomis' unorthodox ideas and practices, though many people tried. Dr. Loomis would always win a debate. Dr. McCaffrey identified with Dr. Loomis, this different, brilliant man.

When the course at Logan was finished, Dr. McCaffrey approached Dr. Loomis about continuing to study with him. Dr. Loomis invited him to Wisconsin to take some of the classes he was teaching there to doctors who wanted to learn how to use the enzyme treatments he had developed.

Dr. McCaffrey jumped at the chance, and for the remainder of his time at Logan, he made regular trips to Wisconsin from St. Louis to study with Dr. Loomis. When he finished school and went into practice in Illinois, Dr. McCaffrey continued to make routine calls to Dr. Loomis to ask him questions when the need arose. One of those phone calls led to a fundamental change in Dr. McCaffrey's work as a healer.

Dr. McCaffrey graduated from Logan in 2000. He worked for a year with an applied kinesiology group and then quickly moved on to opening his own private practice in the Springfield, Illinois, area. Short on money as he was, he had the audacity and confidence to set up two offices right away, one office in Springfield itself, the other in Hillsboro, a nearby rural town.

The Springfield office was suitably spartan. It was one room, and the only piece of furniture in it was an adjusting table. He had no secretary, no desk, and no phone. The office did have windows, and he also kept a small library of medical books there.

(I wonder what Dr. McCaffrey's first patients thought when they walked into that spare office the first time! Did any of them politely back their way out after they took a quick look around?)

At the beginning, there were times during the day when Dr. McCaffrey had no patients. He passed those hours reading medical books. But it sounds like things weren't really all that desperate. Dr. McCaffrey remembers making $7,500 in his first month of practice—not too bad for a chiropractor fresh out of school in 2000 with almost no overhead.

From the very get-go, Dr. McCaffrey drew patients to his practice by starting a show on the local radio station. When he was at Logan, one of his patients owned several radio stations. This man told Dr. McCaffrey that he thought he was charismatic, and that he would do well to start a radio program in which he could talk to thousands of people at a time about health care and his work.

Dr. McCaffrey had never thought of doing a radio show, but it seemed like a good idea. He started his show as soon as he set up his practice in Springfield.

At first, the show wasn't a huge success. "It was crickets," Dr. McCaffrey explained in his colloquial, Midwestern English (as in, it was so quiet you could hear the crickets). Nobody was calling in, and probably not too many people were listening.

As time passed, though, things changed for the better, and calls began to come in. Lots of them. In fact, his show became so successful that the local hospital decided to do a show to compete with Dr. McCaffrey!

## M.E.N. ARE THE CAUSE OF ALL DISEASE

They weren't about to lose any business or prestige to this young whippersnapper of a chiropractor who was not, in their eyes, really a doctor. They started doing a show in the hour right before Dr. McCaffrey's show.

One day, as Dr. McCaffrey was driving into town to do his show, he was listening to the hospital's show. There were two doctors on the show that day: a cancer doctor (an oncologist) and a specialist in lung disease (a pulmonologist).

These physicians were discussing lung cancer and trumpeting the latest advances in the treatment of lung cancer. They talked about how the five-year survival rate for lung cancer was getting better and better, and that now it was up to 12.5 percent.

When Dr. McCaffrey got to the studio, he started his program by questioning why the two doctors in the previous hour hadn't talked about "the six-, seven-, or even eight-year survival rate." This was a provocative lead, to be sure.

One of the doctors who had just been on the air called in immediately. In anger, he called Dr. McCaffrey a charlatan and a quack!

Dr. McCaffrey listened to him for a while, and then he asked him questions. For openers, he asked the good doctor if he was familiar with the *New England Journal of Medicine*, which is like asking the pope if he's familiar with the Bible. Every doctor in the United States knows and has read the *New England Journal*. It's one of the most important medical journals—if not *the* most important—in the United States.

The doctor on the other end of the line said, "Of course."

Then Dr. McCaffrey said, "You mentioned that the five-year survival rate for lung cancer has been improving, and that as we sit here and talk, it's reached 12.5 percent." Dr. McCaffrey paused, then asked, "Doctor, do you know what the five-year survival rate for lung cancer was in 1950?"

Silence.

Dr. McCaffrey answered the question himself. "According to the *New England Journal of Medicine*, it was 12.5 percent. Are you telling me the five-year survival rate hasn't improved at all over the last 50 years?"

*Click*. The doctor hung up.

This experience was a huge lesson for Dr. McCaffrey, but not for the reason you might think. Yes, he had triumphed and proven, in this one instance, that he knew what he was talking about. Yes, it was also true that after that call, no physician ever called in to tell him he was a quack again.

But another doctor did call in with a different message: "You were right about the five-year survival rates for cancer, but you humiliated that man. If you want to keep practicing as a doctor, you should be respectful and calm down."

Dr. McCaffrey took what this man said to heart. He realized that he could handle things in a more peaceful way, and he resolved to never do that again. However, this moment taught Dr. McCaffrey something else. He began to see that it was the other doctor's compartmentalized learning and narrowed view of how the body works that created the situation. As Dr. McCaffrey puts it, "He simply didn't know what he didn't know." Maybe there was a need to bridge the educational gaps between the healing arts. The lead was beginning to turn into gold.

Dr. McCaffrey had two main tools in his doctor's bag when he first opened his practice in Springfield: the chiropractic techniques he learned at Logan, and the nutrition work he learned from Dr. Loomis. In essence, he was a chiropractor who was using a second basic tool—nutrition—to treat his patients. In keeping with his chiropractic training, he made spinal adjustments to his patients to restore the natural flow of information between the brain and the rest of the body. In keeping with Dr. Loomis' theories of nutrition and digestion, he analyzed his patients' digestive processes and gave them enzymes, proteins, and amino acids as necessary to improve them.

In those first years of practice, Dr. McCaffrey leaned heavily on Dr. Loomis' approach to nutrition. In Dr. McCaffrey's words, "I did Dr. Loomis' work from day one when I got out of school."

Remember that Dr. Loomis' nutrition work was grounded in a detailed understanding of the biochemistry of digestion. Essentially, digestion is a bunch of chemical reactions that break down the food you eat so that it can be delivered to the cells in your body as the specific nutrients that each cell needs. There are chemical reactions that break down your food into smaller molecules in your gut, chemical reactions that transport those smaller molecules out of your gut into your body, chemical reactions that carry the nutrients into the cells where they are supposed to go, chemical reactions inside the cell that make use of the nutrients, and, finally, chemical reactions that take all the waste products created by all these other chemical reactions and remove them from your body. For your body to be healthy, all these nutritional and digestive processes must go smoothly and do what they are supposed to do.

Dr. Loomis compiled a specialized urine test that could determine whether all these digestive processes were being carried out in a healthy manner. This test could tell a doctor if a patient was absorbing and digesting fats and proteins correctly, for example. It could detect whether a patient was getting rid of the waste products of digestion properly, and much more.

This test is the key to diagnosing nutritional problems in Dr. Loomis' work. It tells the doctor whether there are any problems in any of the patient's digestive processes, and it tells you what needs to be fixed often before it is broken.

Dr. McCaffrey had great respect for Dr. Loomis' work and adopted his entire approach to nutrition, including the urine test. Over time, though, Dr. McCaffrey altered his understanding of Dr. Loomis' urine test and created his own version of it, which he called the integrated urinalysis panel (IUP).

In those first years of his practice, Dr. McCaffrey was frequently on the phone with Dr. Loomis, asking questions: What does this test result mean? What's wrong with this patient? I followed your instructions, and it didn't work. Why didn't it work?

In the process, he also got to know Dr. Loomis' assistant, Dr. Dennis Frerking, and they developed a fertile telephone relationship as well. It was Dr. Frerking who explained the many aspects of Dr. Loomis' work to Dr. McCaffrey. "Had it not been for Dennis' friendship and mentoring of me," Dr. McCaffrey notes, "I can't even begin to think how lost I would've been in Howard's work." Through Dr. Frerking's guidance, Dr. McCaffrey advanced his knowledge of healing years beyond where it should have been at that point in his career. As Dr. Frerking mentored our young Dr. McCaffrey, he pointed him in new directions. He fostered the idea to constantly question things and to continuously search for answers.

Dr. McCaffrey had much success with his patients in those first few years, but as time passed, he also realized that he was, in his own words, "getting his ass kicked a lot." There were patients that he was unable to help with the two basic tools he was using, and it bothered him immensely.

Things finally came to a head for Dr. McCaffrey while he was treating a patient with liver cancer. When he came to Dr. McCaffrey, the patient had already received and was still receiving standard oncological treatment for his cancer. Dr. McCaffrey worked with him for 19 months, and, in his eyes, the patient was doing extremely well. The patient felt much better. His cancer seemed to be in remission.

Then, in an abrupt change of course, several metastases were found, and, six short weeks later, the patient was gone.

Dr. McCaffrey was puzzled. He was five years out of school. He had done everything he had been taught to treat the patient—everything he learned from both Logan and Dr. Loomis. The patient had gotten remarkably better, but then all of a sudden something changed and the patient died.

Dr. McCaffrey called Dr. Loomis and told him what happened. He told Dr. Loomis that he had followed his instructions to a T, and he asked him why this patient who had been doing so well had worsened all the sudden and died.

Dr. Loomis' response, as I have understood it from Dr. McCaffrey, was this: In his own experience, what happened with Dr. McCaffrey's patient was not unusual. He said that he himself had the exact same experience many times while treating patients who were also receiving chemotherapy and radiotherapy.

They would do extremely well for a spell under his care, and then there would come a time when they would take a sharp turn for the worse and die. Dr. McCaffrey asked why this happens, and Dr. Loomis said he did not know.

This sequence of events unsettled Dr. McCaffrey, and it was to become a turning point in his medical career. He was five years out of school, and there was no doubt in his mind that he wanted to do better for his patients. He decided that if he was going to do better, he was going to have to learn more. He didn't know what that "more" was going to be yet, but he was determined to find it. As the universe would have it, soon thereafter, several new doors opened for Dr. McCaffrey.

Barely two months later, a patient named William came to see Dr. McCaffrey. William had previously had a lymphoma, and after a successful course of treatment with Dr. Donald Kelly, his lymphoma went into remission and had not returned. It had been 11 years.

Dr. Kelly was an orthodontist who developed a well-known means of treating cancer with enzymes, and it was this enzyme treatment that brought William's cancer into remission.

William came to see Dr. McCaffrey all the way from St. Louis because he was looking for another doctor who knew how to use enzymes. His success with Dr. Kelly gave him a great deal of faith in the power of enzyme treatments.

He was looking for a new enzyme doctor because Dr. Kelly had passed away since William first saw him for his cancer. William was now having gastrointestinal (GI) problems, and when he heard that Dr. McCaffrey knew how to use enzymes, he sought him out. Dr. McCaffrey was able to help William with his GI problems, but he got much more than money in return.

Dr. McCaffrey believed in the efficacy of the pioneering enzyme work he learned from Dr. Loomis, but, at this point in his career, he felt he needed to learn more about enzymes. The enzyme treatments he learned from Dr. Loomis didn't always work as well as he would have liked.

Before treating William, Dr. McCaffrey hadn't heard of Dr. Kelly and his enzyme treatment for cancer, so when William mentioned that Dr. Kelly had cured his lymphoma, Dr. McCaffrey decided to learn more about his work. (Remember, it was Dr. McCaffrey's inability to help the patient with liver cancer that led him to resolve that he needed to learn more.)

Given that Dr. Kelly had passed away, Dr. McCaffrey looked for Dr. Kelly's students. He found one who was more than a little interested in passing on what she learned from Dr. Kelly. Her name was Pamela McDougall, and she lived in Idaho. Dr. McCaffrey contacted her, and she offered to give him a course in Dr. Kelly's work if he could get himself to Idaho. She was more than qualified to give that course because she had studied with Dr. Kelly for 17 years!

Dr. McCaffrey lassoed another physician, a friend from California, into coming to take the course with him. They met up in Idaho, and together they took the course from Pamela. The course ended up nudging Dr. McCaffrey's approach to dealing with cancer in a new direction, but it wasn't because he adopted Dr. Kelly's enzyme treatment.

In addition to teaching Dr. McCaffrey about Dr. Kelly's enzyme work, Pamela emphasized the important role emotions play in the causation of cancer. She even brought patients of her own into class to illustrate the concept.

This was not a new idea for Dr. McCaffrey. He had been exposed to this notion before, but hearing it from Pamela at this point in his career brought it to the foreground for him. He decided to take emotions seriously as a cause of illness. Even though Pamela awakened Dr. McCaffrey to the importance of emotions, her technique for dealing with them wasn't exactly earth-shattering. She encouraged her patients to talk about their feelings and emotions and bring them to the surface, all of which is good, but it's rare that simply talking about emotions will clear them from a patient's body. Although Dr. McCaffrey didn't learn a technique for clearing emotions from a patient's body from Pamela (that would come later), studying with Pamela crystalized for him the very important realization that emotions do play a prominent role in causing both cancer and other physical illnesses as well. It dawned on Dr. McCaffrey that what was missing from his medical repertoire was the ability to diagnose and treat bodily illnesses caused by emotional stresses. This was where his next round of growth was going to occur. This was what he had to learn now.

Dr. McCaffrey wasn't driven to learn more because he wasn't doing well with his patients. At this point in time, he was having a good deal of success with his patients, but it was also clear to him that there were lots of patients with whom he could do better, especially those who had somatic illnesses caused by the emotions.

With this understanding in place, Dr. McCaffrey entered a period of several years in which he consciously explored a number of different systems for diagnosing and treating somatic illness caused by the emotions. There were—and still are—lots of different systems floating around, and Dr. McCaffrey set out to discover if any of them really worked. He looked at and experimented with several.

The first system he explored was acupuncture, which has many different systems. There are five traditional Chinese systems, and then there are a number of modern systems that have been invented by contemporary physicians.

Dr. McCaffrey began to study with a Chinese practitioner of acupuncture named Richard Tan, who lived in southern California. Dr. Tan had developed two of his own systems of acupuncture, and he taught both to Dr. McCaffrey. Dr. Tan was especially talented at treating chronic pain. In Dr. McCaffrey's words, "I once saw him put a single needle into a patient who had severe sciatic pain, and the pain stopped instantaneously."

However, Dr. Tan's system didn't give Dr. McCaffrey the tools he felt he needed to treat the pathogenic emotions, so he kept searching.

The next system of treating emotions that Dr. McCaffrey studied was called "total body modification" (TBM), developed by the late Victor Frank. Dr. Frerking had steered Dr. McCaffrey toward Dr. Frank. He had a tape of Dr. Frank giving a class, and he gave it to Dr. McCaffrey. Little did he know he was opening a Pandora's box for Dr. McCaffrey.

This pattern would repeat itself over and over again in the course of Dr. McCaffrey's growth into becoming a mature healer. Many times Dr. Frerking directed him toward something or someone that would end up having a positive impact on Dr. McCaffrey development as a healer.

Dr. Frank was a legendary healer and an accomplished academic. He was a Doctor of Chiropractic, Naturopathic Medicine Doctor, and a Doctor of Osteopathic Medicine. He had been there at the birth of applied kinesiology, a specialized diagnostic tool among chiropractors that involves muscle testing. Dr. Frank had been voted Chiropractor of the Year once, and he was also known to be an enthusiastic healer and intellectual who was full of "piss and vinegar." Most of all, he was open-minded.

After watching the video that Dr. Frerking gave him, Dr. McCaffrey went out to Oakland, California, where Dr. Frank was teaching, to take a class with him. The two became close right away. After that first class, Dr. Frank invited Dr. McCaffrey to postpone his return to Illinois so that he could teach him more. Dr. McCaffrey cancelled his flight.

Over the years, Dr. Frank imparted countless clinical pearls of wisdom. A pivotal lesson Dr. McCaffrey learned from him was to rely on his intuition to diagnose and treat patients. To drive the point home, Dr. Frank told him over and over again, "Forget everything you know and get out of your own way."

At first, Dr. McCaffrey didn't understand what he meant by this. Dr. McCaffrey was busy learning everything he could, and now this man was telling him to forget it all. This couldn't possibly be right. He respected Dr. Frank, though, so he tried to take his injunction to heart. That injunction became an unsolvable riddle—a Zen koan, if you will—that Dr. McCaffrey kept trying to solve.

With the passage of time, Dr. McCaffrey finally cracked the riddle and understood what he meant: Learn everything you possibly can, but when you're with a patient, forget it all and let her rip. Let your intuition tell you how to diagnose and treat your patients. Don't overthink everything. You are not what heals the body. You are merely the tool it chooses to use.

This was an important lesson for Dr. McCaffrey because his background had immersed him in the exceedingly convoluted biochemistry of nutrition.

In truth, Dr. McCaffrey had been relying mostly on reason to arrive at his diagnoses and treatments, and now Dr. Frank was telling him to balance things out by relying on his intuition as well: Fill your tank up with knowledge, then let your intuition guide you when you are actually in the clinic. Be in the moment.

This was another turning point. It was the start of a new and important phase of growth for Dr. McCaffrey, even though he didn't realize it at the time. He had no idea that opening his mind to his intuition—to flashes of insight in the moment—would end up being the first small step in what was to become a period of spiritual growth that would enable him to develop a more profound means of diagnosing and treating his patients. We will return to the next steps in his spiritual growth in a moment.

The second major lesson that Sean learned from Dr. Frank was his system for treating illness caused by emotions, total body modification, mentioned earlier. TBM was a complicated system that Dr. Frank used with "phenomenal" success. It involved 350 different means of diagnosing emotional blockages in the body, and a system for clearing those blocked emotions by balancing energy and electromagnetic fields in a patient's body.

For more than two years, Dr. McCaffrey tried using this system but found that even though Dr. Frank seemed to have incredible success with TBM, he could not reproduce those same results. When Dr. McCaffrey used these techniques, he could help his patients only 40–60 percent of the time. That is, he could lessen a patient's pain 40 percent of the time, or perhaps he could improve the symptoms of a patient's rheumatoid arthritis 60 percent of the time, and so forth.

During this time, Dr. McCaffrey's patients, who had often seen several other doctors without getting better at all, were grateful for the 40–60 percent improvement he provided them. This was far more relief than they had received before, but Dr. McCaffrey wasn't satisfied with this partial success. He kept looking for better means of treatment.

The big breakthrough, the advance that made it possible for Dr. McCaffrey to successfully treat physical illness caused by emotions and to become the extraordinary healer that he is today, unfolded as a series of three events.

The first event occurred when Dr. McCaffrey began to study with another Chinese acupuncturist named Ming Qing Zhu, who works in both China and the United States. He is a sixth-generation acupuncturist, a professor of acupuncture at several Chinese medical schools, and has a private practice based in San Jose, California.

The first thing that struck Dr. McCaffrey about Dr. Zhu was that he had phenomenal success treating patients with neurological diseases and emotional disorders. Dr. McCaffrey had the opportunity to watch Dr. Zhu treat patients, and he saw what can only be described as miracles.

Dr. McCaffrey watched a man who had been paralyzed by a stroke get up and walk after just 20 minutes of treatment. He saw a man who had lost the ability to talk because of Lou Gehrig's disease regain the ability to speak in the course of a weekend.

Dr. Zhu worked these "miracles" by using a method of acupuncture that he himself invented: scalp acupuncture. Traditional acupuncture places needles all over the body. In scalp acupuncture, the doctor places needles only in the scalp to treat diseases of the brain. Dr. McCaffrey learned this method of acupuncture, and he uses it to this day; however, this wasn't the aspect of Dr. Zhu's teachings that led him to his breakthrough.

The breakthrough came when Sean came to terms with one of Dr. Zhu's theories called Dao Yin, which says that there are three elements to making the placement of an acupuncture needle effective: (1) putting the needle in the right place; (2) moving the needle properly once it's in place; and (3) the doctor's intention as they manipulate the needle in the patient's body. The amazing thing about the doctrine of Dao Yin is that it states that the most important element is the doctor's intention. Dao Yin says that proper placement of a needle contributes 10–20 percent to its success. Proper movement contributes another 20 percent, and, finally, the doctor's intention as the needle is placed in the patient's skin and manipulated counts for 60–70 percent of its success.

Think about this for a moment. Would it not seem preposterous to you if a body of research done at Harvard proved that a pediatrician's intention when they gave your child amoxicillin for a lung infection would determine whether the amoxicillin worked? At first glance, it seems absurd.

Nonetheless, this is exactly what the principle of Dao Yin says. The doctor's attitude when they treat a patient is the most important determinant of whether their treatment will work. In Dr. McCaffrey's rendering of the Dao Yin principle, this means, "The doctor has to see the healthy result that he wants to see happen in the patient's body as though it's really happening and has already happened."

Dr. McCaffrey took this principle to heart because it rang a bell for him. It reminded him of something he once read in the notes of his grandfather, the old-school chiropractor. Remember, Dr. McCaffrey's grandfather had known D.D. Palmer, the founder of the field.

The chiropractic taught and practiced by Dr. Palmer around the turn of the 20$^{th}$ century was very different from the chiropractic that is, for the most part, being practiced nowadays, which is, as mentioned earlier, a tame medical practice that limits itself to doing adjustments to the spine to treat back pain, neck pain, and headaches. That's it.

Dr. Palmer's chiropractic saw itself as treating the full spectrum of human illness. Dr. Palmer believed that when he adjusted a patient's spine, he was improving communication between the brain and the rest of the body, and that by restoring that normal communication, he could cure many different types of illness.

More than that, Dr. Palmer also believed that it was important to work with and through a patient's mind to help them. He believed that a basic principle of disease was that negative autosuggestions—negative ideas—could make a person sick. For example, if you believe that you will make yourself sick by going out in the rain, you will indeed come down with a cold. Dr. Palmer believed that he could heal a patient by replacing negative autosuggestions with positive suggestions and allowing the innate intelligence within the body to go to work.

The young Dr. McCaffrey had read about this aspect of Dr. Palmer's work in his grandfather's notes before he met Dr. Zhu. (Early in his career, Dr. McCaffrey's uncle had sent him a large bundle of his father's—Dr. McCaffrey's grandfather's—notes and books, which Dr. McCaffrey had read with great interest.) Now, when confronted with Dr. Zhu's doctrine of Dao Yin, a light bulb went off in Dr. McCaffrey's head. Something about the doctrine of Dao Yin reminded him of the ideas in his grandfather's notes.

Both healers worked directly with their patients' minds to cure bodily illness. Dr. Zhu said that the acupuncturist's intention that he conveyed into his patient's mind while placing acupuncture needles was the most important part of his work. Dr. Palmer worked on the similar premise that a doctor could heal a patient by counteracting negative ideas in the patient's mind.

This connection was the second step in his breakthrough to learning how to treat illnesses caused by emotional stressors.

Inspired by Dr. Zhu, Dr. McCaffrey returned to his grandfather's notes to find out what it was in his grandfather's work that resonated so strongly with Dr. Zhu's Dao Yin doctrine, and he found it—the work of Dr. Thurman Fleet. The late Dr. Fleet was another old-school chiropractor from south Texas who was a close friend of Dr. McCaffrey's grandfather. Legend has it that when Dr. Fleet held office hours, the

M.E.N. ARE THE CAUSE OF ALL DISEASE

Texas Highway Patrol had to control traffic in the area because people lined up for blocks to see him.

Dr. Fleet was a cinematic character who is worth a whole book unto himself. He fought in World War I, and his lungs were destroyed by mustard gas. After years of conventional medical care failed to heal his lungs, he decided that the only way to get better would be to find his own way of healing himself.

One evening in December 1931, Dr. Fleet had an epiphany. For seven days and seven nights he saw things more clearly than he could have ever imagined. In that week, he had visions that gave him the knowledge he needed to heal first himself and then later his patients. Those visions contained massive amounts of knowledge, and that inspired him to write a series of medical books.

In his visions, Dr. Fleet saw that every human being has a mind, body, and soul that are simply energy. Just as Einstein's special theory of relativity says that all matter is energy, Dr. Fleet believed that because our bodies and mind are manifestations of energy, the human mind has the ability to communicate directly with other human minds via a form of energy he called the spirit—the universal spirit.

In other words, just as we use energy in the form of radio waves to transmit television programs, cell phone calls, and internet pages from one place to another, Dr. Fleet realized that it is possible for a person to communicate directly with another person's mind without the two of them talking with one another.

For Dr. Fleet, this was not just philosophical speculation about the nature of the universe. He believed that he could harness the energy/spirit connection between people to heal his patients by communicating directly with the deepest aspects of their mind. And this is exactly what he did. It must have worked well, given that all those patients were lining up outside his office and causing traffic jams.

Dr. Fleet healed his patients by transmitting and embedding positive images of health from his own mind into his patients' unconscious minds. This was the essence of his healing technique: Form a composite personality with the patient and then proceed to treat the body, mind, and soul of the individual.

You have to admit, it does sound an awful lot like Dr. Zhu's idea of transmitting his intention to his patients. Dr. McCaffrey was right in seeing a connection between these two healers' methods.

This all made perfect sense to Dr. McCaffrey, and he immersed himself in Dr. Fleet's work. By the time Dr. McCaffrey discovered Dr. Fleet's work in his grandfather's notes, he was long gone. Luckily for Sean, though, Dr. Fleet left behind extensive writings about how the mind causes bodily illness and how to work with a patient's mind to heal their illness in all those medical books he wrote. Since then, Dr. McCaffrey has read and reread Dr. Fleet's work many times. It became the heart of the McCaffrey Method.

Dr. McCaffrey believes that stress is the cause of all illness, an idea he learned from Hans Selye—the great early scientist of stress—via Dr. Loomis.

Dr. McCaffrey believes three broad categories of stress cause bodily illness: (1) mechanical stress, like breaking a bone or having a gallstone stuck in your gall bladder; (2) emotional stress, like having a bad marriage, being bullied at school, or losing a child or spouse to illness; and (3) nutritional stress, like having too much sugar in your diet or not absorbing fat properly from your gut.

Dr. McCaffrey uses different methods of treatment to clear each type of stress from the body. For example, he uses physical methods of treatment to remove a mechanical stress. This would include the spinal adjustments that are the stock and trade of chiropractic, and muscle memory reintegration (MMR), a system for treating muscle problems that Dr. McCaffrey developed himself.

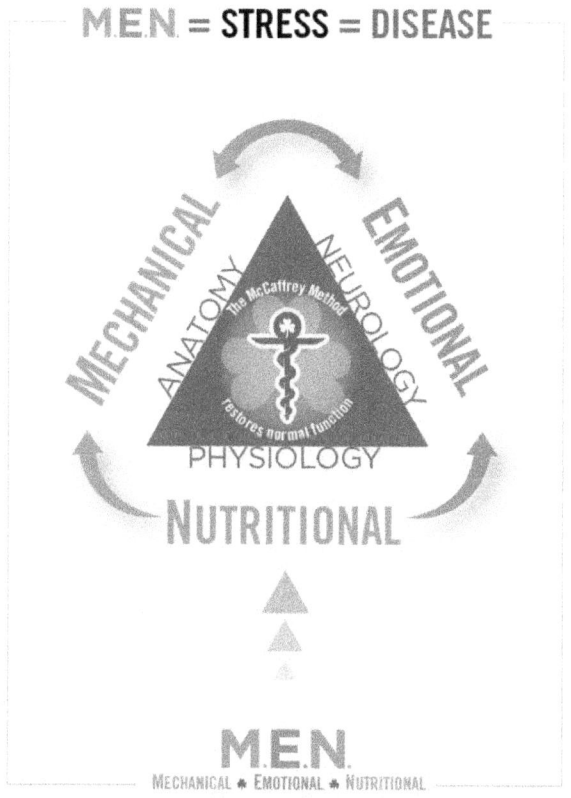

To treat illnesses caused by emotional stress and autosuggestion, Dr. McCaffrey uses two different technologies: (1) He hunts for and helps to clear the stressful emotions from the patient's body; and (2) he embeds positive images of health in their conscious and unconscious mind through suggestion (the work he learned from Dr. Fleet). Ultimately, Dr. McCaffrey believes that most human illness—especially chronic illness—is caused by an emotional stress of one kind or another.

To relieve nutritional stressors, Dr. McCaffrey uses the enzyme and nutritional supplement work he learned from Dr. Loomis: herbal formulas and plants that healing arts from around the globe have used for centuries to combat wounds, infections, and poisonings.

At this point in his career, Dr. McCaffrey uses two fundamental psychological/spiritual tools to diagnose and treat patients with emotional stress: (1) diagnostic epiphanies; and (2) the embedding of positive images of health in a patient's mind.

The diagnostic epiphanies involve receiving information about a patient's body via their actions, words, and mind that clues Dr. McCaffrey into what emotional stressors are causing his patient's illness. Think of it as really honing in on one's intuition and reason.

The embedding of a positive image of health in a patient's mind is a treatment that overpowers the negative ideas and emotions that are causing a patient's illness. Implanting a positive idea sets in motion a myriad of healing processes within a patient's body that return them to health. In Dr. McCaffrey's words, "The image needs to be broad, lawful, logical, and positive to be effective."

If it doesn't seem plausible or scientific that a doctor can heal a patient by communicating directly with their subconscious mind, think of it this way: We have all had the experience of being near a person who is really angry, and we've been able to actually feel their anger. A person's anger can be palpable and contagious. The same is true for the feelings of love and goodness.

It is also possible, in exactly the same way, to tune into a person's subconscious mind if you have the training and the required clarity of mind. This is what Dr. McCaffrey does when he receives diagnostic epiphanies and transmits positive images of health.

The contents of the subconscious mind are subtler than the emotions, and thus more difficult to pick up, but it's the same exact principle. You can feel and hear what's going on in another person's mind because, after all, everything that happens in the mind is created by the movement of electrical impulses in the brain. These impulses are movements of energy that can be detected by scientific instruments or by the human mind. The mind can know the impulses in its own brain as its own thoughts and feelings, or it can sense the impulses in another person's brain as their thoughts and feelings.

All our senses do exactly the same thing: They detect the presence of energy. Our eyes detect the electromagnetic waves that we call light. Our ears detect the air waves that we call sound, and so forth.

Normally, we think of ourselves as having five senses, but we actually have six. This sixth sense is not at all a mystery. Indeed, it's both empirical and something of which we make constant use in our everyday life to be aware of our thoughts, feelings, and emotions. This same sixth sense can also be aware of other people's thoughts, feelings, and emotions.

Dr. Fleet could use this sixth sense to help his patients. By reading and endlessly studying Dr. Fleet's work, Dr. McCaffrey has taught himself how to employ the sixth sense to both diagnose and treat his patients.

The use of diagnostic epiphanies and positive suggestive images of health has become the core of Dr. McCaffrey's healing process—the McCaffrey Method. They are now the most effective aspect of his healing technique.

That does not mean, however, that Dr. McCaffrey no longer does adjustments, acupuncture, or the nutritional work that he learned from Dr. Loomis. Indeed, he uses them all the time to remove the mechanical and nutritional stressors present in his patients' bodies. He continues to treat the "whole body," not just part of it.

He accomplishes three things by clearing these mechanical and nutritional stresses: (1) He gives his patients immediate relief from their symptoms; (2) he shows them that his healing techniques really do work; and, most of all, (3) by removing the mechanical and nutritional stresses, he strengthens the healing effect of the positive images of health and makes it easier for them to work their magic.

Finally, to bring this sketch of Dr. McCaffrey's life as a healer to an end, I should mention that as matters stand now, Dr. McCaffrey has a thriving practice in Springfield, Illinois. Patients come to him from all over the country, and sometimes from even farther away.

In closing, I would like to share one last thing: Dr. McCaffrey asked me to write this book with him for three reasons:

1. He wants people to understand that although mainstream medicine is successful in many respects, it has limitations—especially when it comes to the treatment of chronic illness.

2. He would like people to know that it's possible to heal many of the chronic illnesses that mainstream medicine is unable to treat.

3. He would like to reach out and assist in bridging the gap in healing that would enable other healers and doctors to understand how to integrate their care with one another for the best possible clinical outcomes for their patients.

—Henry Vyner, MD, MA

# CHAPTER 1

# BLOODLETTING, EPIDEMICS, AND THE CHRONIC DISEASES

*"History doesn't repeat itself, but it does rhyme."*

—Mark Twaine

Medicine today is nowhere near what it was in 19th-century America. For one, doctors used barbaric modes of treatment drastically different from anything medicine does today. For example, bloodletting was one of the mainstay treatments of early American medicine, just as it was in both ancient Greece and medieval Europe.

Bloodletting was done in one of two ways. In one method a doctor or barber (really!) would puncture a vein or an artery and allow the blood to gush out of the body. A tourniquet was placed above this patient's elbow, the vein in his forearm was punctured by a lancet, and the blood—flowing under pressure like a geyser—was collected in a bowl.

The other method commonly used to induce blood loss was the application of leeches to the patient's body. The leeches were allowed to dig in and remain there for a good long time while they nourished themselves on the patient's blood—and this was not a rare practice. Thirty-three million leeches were imported into France for medicinal use in the year 1826 alone![1]

---

[1] https://sciencehistory.org/stories/magazine/medicinal-leeches-and-where-to-find-them/

Bloodletting seems barbaric to us now, but for many centuries it was the cornerstone of medical practice in both America and Europe. It was used to treat almost every type of illness: acne, asthma, cancer, cholera, coma, convulsions, diabetes, epilepsy, gangrene, gout, herpes, indigestion, insanity, jaundice, leprosy, plague, pneumonia, scurvy, smallpox, stroke, tetanus, tuberculosis, and many other illnesses as well.

George Washington himself received extensive bloodletting treatments for the illness that took his life, and there has been much speculation among physicians that it was actually the bloodletting that killed him, not his illness. The first president of the United States died immediately after a vigorous round of bloodletting and blistering.

Why in the world did so many physicians—including many physicians considered to be the best doctors of their day—use this brutal, savage procedure to treat their patients? Benjamin Rush, a signer of the Declaration of Independence and the most prominent doctor of the early decades of our republic, was a militant advocate for the use of bloodletting.

The rationale for using bloodletting for medicinal purposes came down to modern European and American medicine from the ancient Greek physicians Hippocrates (460–370 BC) and Galen of Rome (129–216 AD). They both believed that human illness was caused by imbalances of fluids in the body they called the **four humors**.

Today, medicine believes that things like bacteria, viruses, fungi, cigarette smoking, fatty diets, bad genes, and alcoholism cause illness. But from the time of ancient Greece and Rome and lasting well into the 19th and even into the beginning of the 20th century, most European and American doctors practiced medicine based on the idea that the primary causes of illness were imbalances in the four humors.

The humoral theory of disease was the idea that four humors in the human body—blood, phlegm, black bile, and yellow bile—determine whether a person is healthy. The basic belief at the core this theory was that too much or too little of one of the humors would cause illness. An excess of phlegm, for example, was thought to cause bronchitis and pneumonia. An excess of blood was thought to cause dysentery (with its bloody diarrhea) and nosebleeds. It was pretty literal stuff.

The diagnostic task of the doctors operating within the four-humor system was to figure out which humor was out of balance and then take measures to restore it to its proper place. Bloodletting was the technology used by one and all to restore the balance of blood within the body, and it did so by removing what was thought to be excess blood. (Physicians were also not at all timid about bloodletting. Their general rule of thumb was that a patient should be bled until they were just about ready to pass out.)

The rationale and justification for bloodletting came from Galen's humoral theory of illness, and it rested on two misconceptions. The first was that Galen believed that blood was constantly being created and used up by the body. He believed further that blood became useless after its ingredients were consumed, so the body had to keep manufacturing blood to meet its needs.

Galen's second misconception was that the used-up blood would, if left in the body, accumulate and stagnate, causing disease. He didn't understand that our blood is constantly circulating and constantly being cleansed and replenished as it goes. At the time, no one understood this. Science didn't discover circulation until the 17$^{th}$ century, long after Galen. It was discovered by William Harvey, who, when he wasn't doing research, was doctor to the King of England.

With this theory in mind, medicine imagined a remedy for all those illnesses thought to be caused by the accumulation of stagnating blood: bloodletting. This practice seemed to be the obvious way to remove excess, depleted blood from the body. Unbelievable as it may seem now, this idea persisted in America, in some quarters, until the early 20$^{th}$ century.

Bloodletting and the humoral theory of medicine lasted as long as they did because Galen's theories about medicine were supported by the Catholic church. You took your life in your hands if you challenged any of Galen's ideas. Just as the church punished Galileo for claiming that the Earth wasn't the center of the universe, a physician could get in serious trouble for disagreeing with Galen.

Indeed, William Harvey himself watched his medical practice dwindle down to half of what it once had been after he published his theory that the blood of the human body circulates through the body over and over again. His theory was deemed heretical simply because it differed from Galen's conception of the heart and its function. In this climate, Galen's ideas remained influential well into the 18th century, and the practice of bloodletting survived even longer. Old dogmas and habits die hard.

A second difference between American medicine today and American medicine in the 18th and 19th centuries is that early American medicine wasn't effective. Indeed, it was powerless in the face of the epidemics sweeping the nation. Smallpox, diphtheria, yellow fever, and cholera rambled through and decimated America in the 18th and 19th centuries. Science hadn't yet made the discoveries needed to halt them.

Charles E. Rosenberg, a historian of science at Harvard, described the effects of the diphtheria epidemic that laid waste to New England in the early 18th century:

"Perhaps the most dismaying of 18th-century epidemics in America was the outbreak of diphtheria that swept through small towns and villages in northern New England in the 1730s. … In some of the towns, nearly half of the children died, and at times it was feared that the disease would actually destroy the colonies."[2]

Clearly, the destructive power of the epidemics affected the way people saw their lives and their futures, and this persisted until the discovery of antibiotics and vaccines brought the epidemics to a halt.

The epidemics in America weren't limited to New England. Yellow fever devastated Philadelphia in 1793. Cholera roamed the streets of New York and Cincinnati in 1832. The plague ravaged San Francisco at the turn of the 19th century. Infectious disease epidemics were everywhere, and medical science did not yet know how to prevent or stop them because they didn't know what caused them.

For example, the cholera epidemics of the time were said to be caused

---

[2] https://www.researchgate.net/publication/5583432_Siting_Epidemic_Disease_3_Centuries_of_American_History_

by: (1) foul concentrations of air called *miasmas*, a theory used in medieval Europe to explain the bubonic plague; (2) filthy living conditions among the poor blacks and Irish; and (3) the sinful behavior of particular population groups, said to raise the just wrath of an angry God. The religion of the Irish immigrants was said to be an especial culprit in this regard. No mention was made of the *Vibrio cholerae*, the bacteria that causes cholera.

Of course, these theories were incorrect, and they could not possibly have led to any sort of medical action that would have prevented or cured any of the infectious diseases making their way through America more or less unchecked.

Given that mainstream medical science wasn't working; given that the medical practices of the day could not, for the most part, relieve suffering but instead caused it; and given that the medical care system was unable to save people from epidemics and death, several different schools of medical practice took root in America, each one claiming to be the best: the mainstream doctors, the herbalists, the homeopaths, the eclectics and more.

Why were there so many schools of medical practice? Because mainstream doctors weren't really helping their patients, different schools of medical practice sprang up, claiming that they were able to help patients where mainstream medicine couldn't. The different schools of medicine competed with one another to claim the crown of medical competence in America.

Historian of American medicine E. Richard Brown, who was at one time the president of the American Public Health Association, refers to these different schools of medicine in America as "sects." Each sect had their own theory of the causes of disease, and their own distinctive means of treatment.

The main and most prestigious sect of medical practitioners in 19th-century America—the mainstream doctors—was composed of two very different groups: (1) doctors who learned their trade in an apprenticeship; and (2) doctors who had studied at elite medical schools in Europe.

At the beginning of the century, the bulk of American doctors got their medical training as apprentices, learning their trade by working with established doctors. They not only watched their mentors work and learned what they knew, they also helped, mixing medicines and lending an extra hand to help with procedures.

Those who could afford it went overseas to study. The most popular destination for getting a medical education was Edinburgh. At any given time, doctors trained in Europe totaled only about 100 souls. In addition, only three universities—Harvard, Pennsylvania, and Dartmouth—offered medical courses to give apprentice-trained doctors additional training. The Edinburgh-trained doctors and the doctors who received supplemental education at Harvard, Pennsylvania, and Dartmouth formed the elite of American medicine. They were the most prestigious doctors, and they could charge the highest fees for their services.

The elite doctors and the more pedestrian, apprentice-trained doctors were the mainstream doctors of 18th- and 19th-century medicine in America. This was the dominant sect of medical practitioners in early America.

The elite and the apprenticed doctors were united by the fact that they practiced medicine the same way. They all used the same technologies to treat their patients: bloodletting, purgation via the induction of violent vomiting, and the induction of blisters. Sometimes a patient received all three treatments at once. These painful techniques were virtually the entire repertoire of medical treatments in mainstream American medicine throughout the 18th and 19th centuries—although there was one other standard treatment.

Patients would often be weakened by the loss of blood, violent vomiting, and pain inflicted upon them by their doctors. The remedy these doctors applied to their exhausted patients to revive them was a stiff dose of arsenic, given as a tonic to restore the patient's vigor. Arsenic!

Clearly medicine hadn't yet reached its scientific phase.

For the most part, this sadistic brand of medicine was practiced in the cities and large towns of early America, where doctors could find the most patients and make the most money. However, most Americans still lived in either small towns or in rural areas in the country. There were virtually no regular doctors practicing in their midst, so they mostly depended upon herbalists for their medical care. The herbalists were the second sect of medical practitioners in America.

Most herbalists were laypeople who had no formal medical training. Like the mainstream doctors, they learned their trade by doing an apprenticeship, in this case with another herbalist.

Often respected and trusted by their patients, herbalists could help with minor illnesses and relieve some types of pain. Most of all, they didn't inflict upon their patients the painful, humiliating treatments that were the stock and trade of the mainstream doctors of the day—the dreaded bloodletting and all the rest.

A third sect of healers in early America were the homeopaths. Homeopathy was brought to America in 1825 by Hans Birch Gram, a student of Hahnemann, the founder of homeopathy. By 1900, there were 22 homeopathic colleges and 15,000 homeopathic practitioners in the United States. This was a thriving profession.

Homeopathic doctors were trusted and sought out by American patients because, like the herbalists, their treatments were much milder than the devastating treatments of the mainstream doctors. If nothing else, homeopathic patients often got better simply because they weren't left prostrate by the regular doctors' bloodletting and purgation.

One more sect of medical practice popular in the United States was eclectic medicine, a mixture of herbal medicine and physical therapy.

In this climate of competing medical sects, a climate defined by the fact that none of the sects were routinely successful in helping their patients, there was avid competition for patients and prestige. If one of the sects had been visibly and dramatically more successful than the others, there probably would not have been any competition. Everyone would have simply gone to the successful sect for treatment, and that would have been that. (Indeed, this is what happened in the early 20$^{th}$ century with the advent of scientific medicine.) But since none of the sects could consistently relieve their patients' suffering, a free-market competition for market share sprung up between the different sects, or schools, of medical care.

The mainstream doctors tried to dominate the market. They felt it was their right to monopolize American medical care. They were constantly trying to delegitimize and eliminate the other schools of medicine—an idea that continues to this day.

First, in the early 19$^{th}$ century, they tried to forge a monopoly to make it impossible for the herbal healers to practice medicine by systematically persuading state governments to pass laws that restricted and even prohibited the practice of herbal medicine. This attempt was initially successful, but by the middle of the century, it had failed for one simple reason: The American people didn't have confidence in the mainstream doctors because their system of care really didn't work that well. If the majority of people had trusted mainstream medicine, they might have accepted the elimination of the herbalists, but people resisted the attempt to rid the country of herbal healers. The Popular Health Movement arose in America, and by 1850, it had gotten most of the licensing laws repealed.

With the failure of this licensing tactic, the sects continued to compete and began building their own new schools. The idea was that if you could people the landscape with more of your own type of doctor, you could control the market. Then your sect would become the most prominent, most successful medical faction in the field.

Four hundred new medical schools were founded between 1800 and 1900, most of which were private businesses run for profit. Today, there are only 141 medical schools in America.

By the end of the 19$^{th}$ century, there were so many doctors in the United States that there was one physician for every 568 patients.

Whereas in Germany, which was at that time the bastion of the new scientific methods revolutionizing medicine, the average was much lower: only one doctor for every 2,000 people.

This proliferation of medical schools ended up giving mainstream doctors the dominant position in American society. By 1860, regular doctors far outnumbered doctors from all the other sects. There were 10 regular doctors for every other kind of doctor in America.

Still, the medicine practiced by regular doctors was neither roundly respected nor beloved, so the competition between the sects continued, much to the chagrin of mainstream doctors who wanted absolute control of the medical market in America. They wanted a monopoly, and their plan was to get it by controlling access to medical legitimacy.

At the turn of the 19th century, the success and dominance that mainstream doctors wanted finally came to them. They gained that supremacy by doing two very specific things: (1) They took up the practice of the new scientific medicine; and (2) they did some very crafty political maneuvering.

Science began to enter the domain of medicine as early as the 16th century. However, the early discoveries that laid the foundation for the creation of the wondrous medicine we have today were incredibly modest. When you compare them to the discoveries that medicine has made over the last century, they seem like almost nothing. Nonetheless, they were very important because without them, medicine wouldn't be what it is today.

The following is a list of some of the founding discoveries of modern medicine. We'll start with a theory constructed by **Hippocrates**:

1. Hippocrates came up with the theory that illness is caused by natural factors, as opposed to the idea that illness is caused by the gods, the prevailing notion of his time. This groundbreaking move was the first step toward developing a scientific medicine. Even so, Hippocrates' theory of the natural causes of illness—the four-humor theory—was very unscientific.

2. Flemish doctor **Andreas Vesalius** made a second major step forward in the 16th century. He used genuine scientific observations to map out the real anatomy of the body. This was science.

   Before Vesalius, Galen's ideas had dominated the European practice of medicine and its vision of the body. For example, Galen said that the heart had only two chambers, and that blood passed between those two chambers by moving through tiny pores in the fleshy septum that divided them.

   Vesalius dissected and looked at hearts, and he found—as we all know today—that the heart has four chambers and that the blood goes from the right ventricle to the left ventricle by passing through the lungs, where it picks up oxygen.

3. Vesalius' clear depiction of the organs laid the groundwork for the next big step forward. Even though Hippocrates had given birth to the idea that illness is caused by natural factors, it took medicine another 22 centuries to understand that human illness is caused by diseases of the organs. Medicine had not, for example, realized that a heart attack is caused by a malady of the heart, or that the symptom of jaundice is most often caused by a disease of the liver or gallbladder.

   The breakthrough discovery that diseases are caused by abnormalities of the organs was finally made in the 18th century by Italian physician **Giovanni Morgagni**. He did an immense series of more than 700 autopsies, and in 1761 he published his findings. His major discovery was that a patient's symptoms were often correlated with the pathology of specific organs.

   For example, if a patient had been yellow at death (that is, they had been jaundiced), and if they also had a swollen belly filled with fluid (called *ascites* by medicine), they would often have a disease of the liver at autopsy. Or if a patient was found to have a clot in an artery in the lung at autopsy, it was likely the patient had shortness of breath, chest pain, and a cough that produced blood.

In other words, the symptoms of jaundice and ascites were correlated with the presence of a diseased liver; and the symptoms of shortness of breath, chest pain, and a cough that produced blood were correlated with a clot in an artery in the lung.

Morgagni realized that this meant that diseased organs caused human illness, grasping the idea that there was a correlation between organs and symptoms. We take this idea for granted now, and, indeed, it's the foundation of modern medicine. In the middle of the 18<sup>th</sup> century, though, this was a new, mammoth step forward.

4. Another crucial step forward in understanding the cause of disease came with the discovery that diseases of the organs were actually diseases of the cells of the organs. This discovery was made by the remarkable German scholar and scientist **Rudolph Virchow** in the middle of the 19<sup>th</sup> century. Morgagni had recognized that illness is caused by the body's organs, but Virchow took his work one step further.

Consider this: Lung cancer is defined as the presence of cancer cells in the lung, whereas bacterial pneumonia is defined as the presence of bacteria and inflammatory fluid in the cells of the lung. With this discovery, scientists realized that different diseases are caused by, and also defined as, specific cellular abnormalities in the organs. This discovery is now one of the fundamental principles of modern medicine.

We need to step back now for a moment and recognize something about this list of early medical discoveries. Although these revelations were the founding principles of modern scientific medicine, they did not produce—at the time—any advances in the actual practice of medicine. They were fundamental insights into the causes of disease, but they didn't change or improve the treatments that doctors were giving to their patients.

After these discoveries were made, mainstream medicine in America and Europe continued to center around the triad of "heroic" treatments—bloodletting, purgation by vomiting, and blistering. Despite Morgagni's and Virchow's discoveries, physicians continued to use methods mandated by the ancient humoral theory of medicine.

Science did, however, finally begin to have an impact upon the practice of medicine at the end of the 19th century. Discoveries were made that actually led to improvements in the way physicians practiced medicine in their daily work.

The first big breakthrough was the discovery that tiny little animals—animals invisible to the naked eye—cause diseases. Does this sound familiar? It should. Those animals were the bacteria and viruses. Later, other small organisms—fungi, rickettsia, and the protozoa—would be discovered to also cause disease.

With this discovery, medicine began to understand that the epidemics regularly sweeping across continents and decimating large swathes of the population were caused by these tiny organisms. And this was just the beginning.

Medicine turned a corner with the first groundbreaking discoveries of French scientist Louis Pasteur, who made his name by saving the French wine industry from a viral infection of its grapes. He went on to give us pasteurization, and he also invented the first viable treatment for rabies.

These discoveries created the new field of microbiology, and the findings of this new field were different from the earlier findings of scientific medicine in one crucial respect: They actually improved medical care.

The science of microbiology held out the prospect of developing straightforward methods that could be used to both prevent and treat infectious diseases. They also led to the widespread use and acceptance of antiseptic surgery, vaccination, and public sanitation.

Prior to the 20th century, infectious diseases were the leading causes of death in both Europe and America. The epidemics they caused routinely killed large swathes of people. The bubonic plague epidemic of the late 14th century is thought to have killed somewhere between 25 and 50 percent of all the people living in Europe at that time.

With the discovery that bacteria and other microorganisms caused infectious diseases, humanity realized that it was going to be possible to do something about these epidemics, that science would be able to find the culprits causing these frightening epidemics. This was a huge sea change, both scientifically and psychologically.

In 1883 and 1884, Edwin Klebs and Friedrich Loeffler found the germ that causes diphtheria. Then Emil von Behring and his colleagues produced a diphtheria antitoxin in the 1890s. Progress was on the horizon.

As a result, people began to believe that medicine would be able to protect them from infectious diseases and epidemics. Life was going to change for the better. The discovery that microorganisms were causing the epidemics instilled a great deal of optimism in both the medical profession and the general public.

## MAINSTREAM MEDICINE AND SCIENCE

In America, mainstream medicine moved to take proprietary possession of scientific medicine. Mainstream doctors began to practice scientific medicine and to define themselves as such.

The momentum toward scientific medicine picked up when Johns Hopkins Medical School in Baltimore, Maryland, the first medical school devoted to the teaching of scientific medicine, was founded in 1893. Soon thereafter, Harvard, Yale, and the University of Pennsylvania medical schools followed suit, hiring Hopkins graduates to teach in their schools.

At the same time, country doctors were, for the most part, skeptical of the virtues of scientific medicine and continued to practice the same style of medicine they always had.

With the adoption of scientific medicine, doctors practicing mainstream medicine became competent and successful. Now that they were truly helping their patients, people began to respect and trust them. The general public was more willing to accept mainstream doctors as the sole practitioners of medicine. With the wind in their sails, mainstream medicine sought to develop a monopoly over American medicine, a monopoly established by the work of the American Medical Association (AMA).

In all fairness to the AMA, they wished to establish a monopoly over American medicine for a mixed bag of reasons. First, they simply wanted to increase the prestige and income of their doctors—the mainstream and increasingly scientific doctors of America.

As time passed, though, a second, more noble reason arose. Mainstream doctors genuinely wanted to improve the quality of medical care in America. It wasn't just money driving the AMA to take control of medical education and licensing in America.

Founded in 1847, the AMA's goal from the very beginning was to reform American medicine by giving its doctors a monopoly over the practice.[3] At first, it wasn't successful. By the end of the century, the AMA was just a sleepy little organization with no real power and only 8,000 members.

Things changed in 1901 when the AMA was taken over by reformists who championed the practice of scientific medicine. The reformists completely reorganized the AMA, merging all the country's local and state medical societies into the AMA itself.

With this move they launched a concerted effort to gain control of medical licensing boards in all the states. With control of the boards, they could determine who could and could not be a doctor. Thus energized, the AMA began to attract attention, and by 1910, its membership swelled to 70,000.

---

3 https://www.ama-assn.org/about/ama-history/ama-history

Licensing was not, however, the only measure that the AMA took to gain control of American medicine. In 1904, the AMA created the Council on Medical Education (CME) whose explicit goal was to exercise control over medical education. Their plan was to improve medical care by making all medical schools teach the new scientific medicine.

To this end, the CME designed an ideal medical school curriculum, one in which a student would first study for two years the basic sciences upon which medicine was based—anatomy, physiology, pathology, and pharmacology—followed by two years of clinical study in a teaching hospital. This meant that a medical school had to possess a teaching hospital in which students could get their clinical training. At that time, most schools didn't have teaching hospitals, although it's standard procedure now.

Building the teaching hospitals would require large sums of money, and someone was going to have to pay for their construction. In later years, the robber baron industrialists would bankroll the building of the new scientific medical schools and their teaching hospitals.

With their blueprint in place, the CME surveyed all 166 medical schools in America to evaluate whether they matched their blueprint. Many did not, and, as a result, several medical schools closed their doors right away. Within three short years the number of medical schools dropped from 166 to 131, but this was just the beginning. There were more evaluations to be done and more pruning to come.

Empowered and emboldened by this first success, the AMA reached out to and formed a working relationship with the Carnegie Foundation for the Advancement of Teaching, which was, of course, funded by Andrew Carnegie's steel money. The AMA sought the help of the Carnegie Foundation because they thought that a study of medical schools by the foundation would lend an aura of objectivity to the evaluations that the AMA had already done. After all, the AMA was a biased sectarian medical organization, and they realized it would help their cause if an "objective" institution evaluated America's medical schools and reached the same conclusions.

In addition, the AMA also hoped that the Carnegie Foundation would lend prestige and money to their efforts to shape and transform American medical education. In particular, the AMA realized it was going to take a great deal of money to fund the building of the scientific laboratories, full-time faculties, and teaching hospitals that the new scientific medical schools would require. The AMA thought they could attract a new source of funding—wealthy industrialists—by working with Carnegie and the Carnegie Foundation.

The CME proposed to the Carnegie Foundation that it do a study of the quality of American medical schools, which the foundation agreed to do, choosing Abraham Flexner to head up the study. Abraham was the brother of physician Simon Flexner, the director of the Rockefeller Institute for the study of medicine. The deck was stacked. (Flexner would later play a crucial role in bringing Rockefeller money to the new scientific medical schools that were recommended by the Flexner Report.)

Flexner took 18 months to do his study. During those months, he personally visited all the medical schools in both Canada and the United States, which means he averaged three and a half days per school—including traveling time. In 1910, Flexner issued a report on his findings (called the Flexner Report), which had a major impact on medical education and the practice of medicine in the United States.[4]

When Dr. Vyner, who introduced this book, was in medical school, he was the only student representative on the faculty curriculum committee whose job it was to evaluate and recommend changes to the curriculum as needed. The Flexner Report came up frequently in those discussions, and it was spoken of with great reverence.

The report criticized much of what was going on in American medical schools, taking particular aim at the fact that most medical schools were simply businesses that weren't part of a larger university. People were admitted to these commercial medical schools if they had the money.

This was true. For-profit medical schools admitted as many students as possible because it increased their earnings. Little attention was

---

4 https://daily.jstor.org/the-1910-report-that-unintentionally-disadvantaged-minority-doctors/

paid to the merits of entering students, even though they were going to become the next generation of doctors taking care of the American people. Flexner justly and harshly criticized all of this.

He also criticized the general lack of scientific education in the medical schools of the day. At the time of the Flexner Report, only a few medical schools were following the Johns Hopkins model of scientific medical education.

Ultimately, Flexner decided that most medical schools were substandard. He divided the schools he visited into three categories based on how good he thought they were.

The first group, which was small, was composed of schools that were successfully following the Hopkins model. The second group were schools that Flexner judged to be substandard but redeemable if large amounts of money were poured into them. The third misbegotten group were, in Flexner's estimation, schools of such inferior quality, they were beyond redemption. Flexner recommended these schools be shut down—recommendations that were followed. At the time of the report, there were 131 medical schools in the United States. Twenty years later, the number was 76.[5]

In addition, entrance requirements for medical school were tightened up. In 1904, the majority of medical schools (95 percent) required nothing more than a high school diploma to gain entrance. By 1929, all American medical schools required their entrants to have at least two years of college education.[6] (Now, of course, one must have four years of college and a degree to get into a medical school.)

All these changes were for the good, and they improved the quality of medical education; however, they also reduced the number of doctors in America and made it more difficult to obtain a medical education, which was a stated goal of the AMA from the beginning. They thought that a smaller supply of doctors would make them more valuable commodities worthy of a greater income and increased prestige. They were forming an elite class within the population.

---

5 https://en.wikipedia.org/wiki/Medical_school_in_the_United_States
6 https://www.ncbi.nlm.nih.gov/pmc/articles/PMC2967338/

In addition, these new requirements made medicine a profession that was restricted to the sons of wealthy upper- and middle-class families, which was one of Flexner's goals. He thought that making medicine an upper-class profession would help ensure the quality and prestige of the medical profession.

Most of all, the Flexner Report helped the AMA and mainstream medicine eliminate their competitors—the other sectarian medical practitioners. Indeed, the chairman of the AMA's Committee on Medical Education, Dean Bevan, later confessed, "We were, of course, very grateful to ... Flexner" for helping "us to put out of business" the homeopathic and eclectic medical schools. (Walsh, J. J. (1970). *History of the Medical Society of the State of New York*. New York: Medical Society of the State of New York.)

In addition, five black medical schools were deemed inadequate by the Flexner Report, and they too were forced to close down when the Flexner critique dried up their funding. By 1942, there was only one black doctor for every 3,377 black patients.

However, the Flexner Report was beneficial in one very important respect. The principal positive impact of the report was that it engineered the transformation of American medicine. The sectarian landscape of 18th and 19th century medicine was replaced by a health care system in which scientific medicine became the dominant and **only accepted means** of medical care in America.

This was a very positive development because it generated better medical care. With the advent of scientific medicine, yellow fever, typhoid, malaria, and polio were virtually eliminated from the United States. Insulin was discovered, improving the lives of diabetic patients. Life expectancy ballooned. For most of human history, the average human lifespan was less than 50 years. It began to climb in the 19th century, and by 1900 it had risen to 47 in the United States. By 1950, 50 years after the advent of scientific medicine, life expectancy had risen to 69.[7]

---

[7] https://www.verywellhealth.com/longevity-throughout-history-2224054

In addition, surgery became the domain of miracles. We now have kidney and heart transplants, and hip and knee replacements. Surgeons developed the ability to remove fatty deposits from the coronary artery to prevent heart attacks and from the carotid artery to prevent strokes.

Now it's possible to restore sight by replacing a lens with a cataract. We can save a woman's life by removing an ectopic pregnancy. We can save lives by removing a deadly obstruction of the bowel. The list goes on.

With the success of scientific methods, mainstream medicine became an effective, respected institution within American society. People were grateful for the new scientific medicine because they knew that now they could go to a doctor and get better. Pain would be relieved. Diseases would be cured. The days of the traveling medicine shows were over.

## THE CHRONIC DISEASES

This was, of course, all for the good. However, if we're honest with ourselves, the scientific medicine that the Flexner Report bequeathed to us has one **major** clinical shortcoming: chronic diseases. Modern scientific medicine can't cure chronic diseases. That's why they're chronic! They go on and on and become chronic because we can't cure them, and, as we are about to see, they are our largest medical problem.

Take as an example coronary artery disease that causes heart attacks. This chronic disease is the largest killer of people in the United States. It's a disease process in which fats are deposited inside the coronary artery, the artery that brings blood to the heart. This deposition of fats reduces blood flow to the heart, and this causes heart attacks.

Medicine is capable of giving you medications that will slow down the deposition of fats in the coronary artery. The process can even be reversed a bit. If necessary, we can go even further by surgically inserting a tube in the artery that will prop it open and improve blood flow. But we can't cure and bring to a permanent halt the process of fat deposition in the coronary artery (called *atherosclerosis* by medicine). Nor can we stop the deposition of fats in the artery that brings blood to the brain—the carotid artery—which is the main cause of strokes.

Chronic diseases—the diseases we can't cure—are not a small problem. They are the major health problem of all humanity. More than half of all Americans suffer from a chronic disease. In 2005, the number stood at 133 million.[8] Today the number is even higher at around 155m, a staggering 60 percent of all adult Americans with at least one chronic illness.[9] Globally, one in three human beings suffers from **more than one** chronic disease.

Worse than that, every year, 60 percent of all deaths in the world—three out of every five—are caused by chronic diseases.[10] This includes deaths caused by heart disease, stroke, cancer, depression, dementia, diabetes, and the chronic respiratory diseases—most of which are caused by smoking. In the United States, 70 percent of all deaths are caused by chronic diseases.[11]

Given these numbers, we have to conclude that something is dreadfully wrong with our medical care system. It's unable to prevent or cure the chronic diseases causing the majority of our deaths.

The scale of the burden that chronic disease imposes upon America can be gauged by the startling figure that **more than 75 percent of our national health care spending is used to treat patients who have chronic diseases.**[12]

Here are a few of the details of the medical and existential damage that is caused by the chronic diseases in America:

1. **Heart disease is the leading cause of death among Americans, and strokes are the third. Together they cause 30 percent of American deaths every**

---

8 https://stacks.cdc.gov/view/cdc/5509/cdc_5509_DS1.pdf
9 https://www.americanactionforum.org/research/chronic-disease-in-the-united-states-a-worsening-health-and-economic-crisis/
10 https://www.who.int/data/gho/data/themes/topics/topic-details/GHO/ncd-mortality
11 https://www.ncbi.nlm.nih.gov/pmc/articles/PMC5876976/
12 https://www.commonwealthfund.org/publications/issue-briefs/2023/jan/us-health-care-global-perspective-2022

**year**.[13] They are both chronic diseases caused by high blood pressure and atherosclerosis, the deposition of fats on the inside of arteries over long periods of time. These are illnesses we simply don't know how to cure because we don't know what causes them.

2. **Cancer**, America's second leading cause of death, is another chronic disease we can't cure.[14] As of this writing, cancer still **kills half a million people a year**, even though we've made significant advances in the early detection and treatment of cancer.

3. **Thirty-seven million Americans live with diabetes**, and 96 million have pre-diabetes.[15] Diabetes is the leading cause of kidney failure, blindness, and limb amputation for all adults more than 20 years of age. Diabetes also increases the risk of developing heart disease and strokes.

4. Then there's arthritis, the leading cause of disability in America.[16] **One out of every five adults—more than 50 million people—in America has arthritis** that has been diagnosed by a doctor.[17] Arthritis can be both painful and disabling. Perhaps you can't go for a run or a walk because of the pain in your knee from arthritis. Perhaps you can no longer play the piano because you have arthritis of the hands that makes your fingers too stiff. **Nineteen million Americans have to limit their activities because they have arthritis**.

---

13 https://www.cdc.gov/heartdisease/facts.htm
14 https://www.cdc.gov/chronicdisease/resources/publications/factsheets/cancer.htm
15 https://www.cdc.gov/chronicdisease/resources/publications/factsheets/diabetes-prediabetes.htm
16 https://www.mayoclinic.org/diseases-conditions/arthritis/in-depth/arthritis/art-20046440
17 https://www.cdc.gov/arthritis/data_statistics/disabilities-limitations.htm

5. Another chronic disease is obesity. **One in three American adults are seriously obese**, which increases their risk of getting heart disease, hypertension, arthritis, back pain, and diabetes.[18] How did this come to pass in a land of hardy settlers, pioneers, cowboys, and farmers?

6. Finally, **lung diseases** caused by smoking cigarettes—chronic bronchitis and emphysema—**kill more than 90,000 people a year**.[19]

(The figures I listed above all come from two seriously reputable institutions: our Centers for Disease Control and Prevention, an agency of the Department of Health and Human Services; and the World Health Organization.)

Chronic diseases such as these—diseases that modern medicine can't cure because it doesn't yet understand their cause—are the main purveyors of disability and death in the United States. It's that simple, and yet it's difficult to believe that this is happening in the United States of America, a true bastion of excellent medical care in many ways.

Dr. Vyner routinely travels to and works in underdeveloped countries around the world, as he is also an anthropologist. Long ago, it became an article of faith for him that if he ever got seriously (or even moderately) ill out there in the world, he would come back to America to get medical care. Having seen the quality of medical care elsewhere in the world, he realized that far and away the wisest thing to do would be to return home.

And yet, if we're truly honest with ourselves, as both patients and doctors, we have to admit that something is vitally wrong with modern medical care. This is the 21st century, yet seven out of 10 Americans die of illnesses that medicine can neither understand nor cure. It wouldn't be hard to believe that seven out of 10 people in medieval Europe were dying of diseases that couldn't be cured, but it's just about impossible to believe that we can say the same about Americans today.

---

18 https://www.cdc.gov/obesity/data/adult.html
19 https://www.verywellhealth.com/lung-disease-from-smoking-5202555

## M.E.N. ARE THE CAUSE OF ALL DISEASE

The time has come to admit that something is profoundly wrong with modern mainstream medicine. Even though it's capable of doing much that is excellent, modern medicine is helpless in the face of chronic diseases—our most deadly diseases now that infectious diseases have been tamed.

This epidemic of chronic diseases tells us that there must be something fundamental about the diseases of the human body that modern medical science does not yet understand.

With all of this said, there are alternative healers in the United States—and elsewhere—who can cure chronic diseases. Dr. McCaffrey is one of them, and the key to making headway with chronic diseases is to enter into a dialogue with Dr. McCaffrey and his alternative colleagues to find out what they know.

If they really can cure chronic diseases, we have to open ourselves to the possibility that they know something that scientific medicine doesn't. Given mainstream medicine's poor track record with chronic diseases, we must make an honest attempt to determine if there is something to be learned from the healers who are actually able to cure the chronic diseases.

The Flexner Report made scientific medicine the dominant school of health care in America, and, as we know, that did much to improve the quality of medical care in the United States.

At the same time as Flexner and his allies lifted up scientific medicine and put it on the pedestal on which it now stands, they delegitimized all other schools of medical care in America. It wasn't enough for them to simply improve their own brand of medicine. They were set on having a monopoly and destroying any competition—just like the industrialists who funded them.

The Flexner Report created a climate in which it became very difficult—if not impossible—for alternative medical practitioners and their medical schools to get licensed and to get funding. Indeed, it was a stated goal of the AMA to denigrate and eliminate the practice of homeopathy, chiropractic, and other alternative forms of healing.

Given that the scientific medicine bequeathed to us by the Flexner Report is genuinely unable to either understand or cure chronic diseases, the time has come for the self-appointed gods of mainstream medicine to listen to and take an honest look at the alternative healers. The time has come to see what they know that makes it possible for them to cure and even prevent the chronic diseases that end so many lives. It's time to reopen the doors that the Flexner Report closed.

In the next chapter, we'll take a look at how mainstream medicine goes about treating chronic illnesses, and in the chapter after that, we'll examine how Dr. McCaffrey treats and cures those chronic illnesses.

# CHAPTER 2

# CHRONIC DISEASES AND THE EMOTIONS

*"Unexpressed emotions will never die. They are buried alive and will come forth later in uglier ways."*

—Sigmund Freud

In November 2018, a Gallup poll found that 80 percent of Americans think that their medical care is either excellent or good. The percentage is even higher among elderly people (over 65) at 88 percent. In addition, a study done by scientists at Harvard and MIT found that 60 percent of Americans feel confident they'll get the best possible treatment if they get seriously ill and go see a doctor.

We doctors feel the same way about the quality of the medical care we give our patients. We come out of medical school fully believing in the truth of the medicine we've learned and its ability to diagnose and cure disease.

And it's easy to understand why everyone feels this way. Patients really do get better when they go see a doctor. Sometimes the change for the better is so dramatic, it seems as though God has intervened and worked a miracle.

Imagine you have an excruciating pain in your belly that finally gets so bad you have to go to the emergency room to get help. You have no idea what's causing your pain as there are hundreds of causes of belly pain. All you know is that you're hurting and scared; something must really be wrong given how bad the pain is.

Luckily for you, the doctor you see in the emergency room is well trained, serene, and competent; and she immediately find the problem. You have an inflamed appendix. Within half an hour, you're in surgery and on the way to getting well again.

It will almost certainly be the same situation if you have meningitis, pneumonia, a broken bone, or an ectopic pregnancy. When you go see your doctor, you'll receive the right diagnosis and treatment. Modern medicine does a lot of things well.

However, if we dig a little bit deeper, and take an honest look at the health care we receive, it becomes apparent that modern medicine has some serious blind spots, the largest being the illnesses we call chronic.

A chronic illness is an illness we can't cure, and since we can't cure it, it goes on and on. It might last for years, decades, even the rest of a patient's life. High blood pressure (called *hypertension* by doctors) is a disease of the cardiovascular system and a good example of a chronic illness.

The cardiovascular system is composed of the heart, the blood vessels, and the blood that courses through them. The heart is a pump, and it pumps blood to all of the body through a web of flexible pipes we call arteries and veins. Your blood carries oxygen and nutrients to the tissues of your body, and the veins return your blood to your heart and lungs to pick up more oxygen and nutrients along the way. Hypertension (high blood pressure) is a condition in which the pressure of the blood in your arteries is elevated above the normal level.

High blood pressure is dangerous because it causes an immense amount of other very serious medical problems. It can lead to heart attacks, heart failure, strokes, kidney disease, and eye disease. It's called "the silent killer" because it can kill you without you even being aware that it's damaging your body.

## M.E.N. ARE THE CAUSE OF ALL DISEASE

Why, then, is high blood pressure a chronic disease? Because we can't cure it.

"But wait a minute," you might say. "Aren't there medicines that lower blood pressure?" Yes, there are medications that can lower your blood pressure, but they don't cure high blood pressure. You have to take the medicines forever. If you stop taking the medications, your blood pressure will go back up.

If lowering high blood pressure isn't a cure of hypertension, then what does it mean to cure a disease?

We can understand what it means to cure an illness by taking a look at the treatment of a disease we can cure: bacterial pneumonia.

Pneumonia is an infection of the lungs that can be caused by any number of different microorganisms. For example, it can be caused by several different kinds of bacteria, viruses, and fungi, which are the most common causes of an infectious pneumonia. If bacteria is causing your pneumonia, your body will try to protect you by removing the bacteria from your lung by mounting two responses to it: the inflammatory response and the immune response.

Working together, the inflammatory and immune responses flood your lung with white blood cells, fluid, chemicals, and pus that break down, kill, and digest the bacteria. The inflammatory response makes you sick in the process of making you better.

Normally, the lungs are full of nothing but air! This condition in which your lungs are full of liquid and white blood cells is called pneumonia. (The definition of a pneumonia is a hunk of lung tissue that's infiltrated with bacteria, fluid, white blood cells, and pus.)

Medicine is more than capable of curing bacterial pneumonia by killing the bacteria with antibiotics. (Antibiotics are medications that kill or debilitate bacteria.) When the antibiotics kill the bacteria in your lungs, your lungs will return to their normal state in which the air sacs contain only air.

What's more, once the bacteria have been removed from your lung, you no longer need to continue taking the antibiotics. Your lungs will have returned to their normal and healthy state, and they'll stay in that normal state even if you stop taking your medicine. You're cured!

But things are different with high blood pressure—and all the other chronic diseases. Medicine can't cure most cases of hypertension.

If you have what's called **essential hypertension**, one of the two basic types of hypertension, you'll have to take medicine for the rest of your life—the key indicator that you have a chronic disease.

Secondary hypertension, the other basic type of the disease, is a case of high blood pressure for which a cause can be found. Many different types of illness can cause high blood pressure— for example, several kidney and adrenal gland diseases. In secondary hypertension, the high blood pressure is secondary to, or caused by, another disease.

Interestingly, even though many different types of disease can cause high blood pressure, only 5 percent of all cases of hypertension are the secondary type. This means that 95 percent of all cases of hypertension are essential hypertension—high blood pressure for which a biological cause can't be found. Of course, there has to be a cause for essential hypertension, but so far medicine hasn't figured out what it is. Even so, medical science has found ways to lower a patient's blood pressure by intervening in the pathogenesis of essential hypertension.

"What," you might ask, "is the pathogenesis of a disease?" Every disease has a pathogenesis, which is related to, but different from, the cause of a disease. Let's look again at the bacterial pneumonia we discussed earlier.

The cause of bacterial pneumonia is, of course, the bacteria themselves. If the bacteria aren't present in the lung, there will be no pneumonia.

The pathogenesis of bacterial pneumonia is the group of physiological processes that create the pneumonia once the bacteria are present in the lung—the sequence of processes by which the lung becomes filled with inflammatory fluid, white blood cells, and pus.

The basic pathogenetic processes that create bacterial pneumonia are the inflammatory and immune responses that the body mounts when bacteria is present in the lung. They create the pneumonia by bringing white blood cells and fluid into the lungs.

In general, then, the pathogenesis of a disease is the process by which that disease develops, the process by which the cause of a disease is translated into the full-blown disease itself.

When it comes to essential hypertension, we don't know the cause of the high blood pressure, but we do know a great deal about its pathogenesis—about the mechanisms by which the body creates the high blood pressure of essential hypertension. This knowledge allows us to treat and reduce a patient's high blood pressure, but not cure it.

For example, we can reduce a person's blood pressure by giving them a medicine that will reduce their blood volume. This is much the same as reducing the pressure in a tire or a basketball by allowing some of the air to escape—they get soft because the air pressure inside them is reduced. The same thing happens when you reduce the volume of blood inside the cardiovascular system. This is just one mechanism we can use to disrupt the pathogenesis of hypertension and reduce a person's blood pressure.

We can also give a patient a medicine that reduces the amount of **angiotensin** in their blood. Angiotensin is a protein that is naturally present in the body that causes your arteries to constrict, and when your arteries constrict, your blood pressure increases. However, when you reduce the amount of angiotensin in a person's body, their arteries dilate instead and their blood pressure goes down. Angiotensin is one of many mechanisms that the body uses to regulate its blood pressure.

Even though reducing the amount of angiotensin in the blood and reducing the blood volume both disrupt the pathogenesis of high blood pressure, when you treat a disease by obstructing its pathogenesis, you're not removing the cause of the disease. You're not curing it. We don't know how to cure essential hypertension—or any other chronic disease.

In contrast, when you give a person an antibiotic for pneumonia, you remove the cause of the disease—the bacteria. This cures the pneumonia. If, however, you didn't give the patient an antibiotic, but you did give them a medication that dried out their lungs, they would get somewhat—but not entirely—better. They would certainly not be cured. As soon as you stopped giving them the medication that dries out their lungs, full-blown pneumonia would return.

The same is true of essential hypertension. We can give a patient who has essential hypertension medicines to reduce their blood pressure, but as soon as they stop taking their medicine, their blood pressure will increase again because we haven't removed the cause of their hypertension. We can't eliminate the cause of essential hypertension because we don't know what it is.

This means that we give patients with essential hypertension symptomatic treatment. We treat the symptom of high blood pressure by reducing the pressure, and we often do a good job of it. But we're not curing it. This is why essential hypertension is a chronic disease. It goes on and on.

What, then, is the problem? Why are so many of us suffering from, and dying of, diseases that modern medicine doesn't understand? Perhaps the answer is in the mind.

## CHRONIC ILLNESS AND THE MIND

Jean-Martin Charcôt was a well-known, respected French scientist and doctor in the second half of the 19th century. In his day, he carried the honor of being called a "Prince of Science" (French: *Prince de la Science*), which meant that he was seen as both a genius of medical science and a man of ways and means in society. He was powerful and influential in medical circles and a doctor to kings and princes. Roundly regarded as the greatest neurologist of his day, neurological diseases have been named after Charcôt, and some still carry his name. When Dr. Vyner was in medical school, he learned about an illness called Charcôt-Marie-Tooth disease in Europe—Lou Gehrig's disease here in America.

In Charcôt's day, it was generally believed in medical circles that if a patient had a paralyzed arm or leg, it would have been caused by some kind of disease of, or injury to, the central nervous system—the brain, spinal cord, or peripheral nerves. Charcot disagreed. He believed that the mind could also cause a paralysis of an arm or leg, and he did an ingenious series of experiments to prove it.

First, Charcôt showed that a posthypnotic suggestion—nothing more or less than an idea implanted in the mind—could cause the paralysis of an arm. Charcot did this by hypnotizing a patient and giving them the posthypnotic suggestion that when they awoke, their arm would become paralyzed when he slapped them on their back. In other words, a simple idea in the patient's mind caused their arm to be paralyzed—a rather serious physical problem.

What could be more straightforward? With this simple experiment, Charcôt proved that an idea in the mind could cause physical problems in the body!

But Charcôt did not leave it at this. To make his discovery more scientific and to convince the skeptics, Charcôt went one step further. He did a series of experiments that demonstrated that it was possible to unequivocally tell the difference between a biological paralysis and a psychological paralysis. He proved that a paralysis of the arm caused by the mind involves a different set of muscles than a paralysis caused by a biological injury to the brain or a nerve.

Charcôt's work on posthypnotic paralysis was part of a larger vein of clinical research that proved that the mind can actually cause physical illness. Given Charcôt's stature in the worlds of medicine and science, his work gave rise to even more research in this area.

In the second half of the 19th century, medical science was beginning to close in on the notion that fixed ideas in the mind (French: *idée fixe*) could cause both physical and psychological illness. Evidence was beginning to accumulate that these ideas could cause both somatic and psychological symptoms. Much of that evidence was being generated by some of the most famous doctors of the day: Sigmund Freud, Pierre Janet, and Carl Jung.

While Charcôt's research proved that a physical symptom—the paralysis of an arm—could be created by using hypnosis to **implant** an idea in a patient's mind, the work of famed French psychologist Pierre Janet provided a different kind of proof that fixed ideas can cause physical illness. He showed that he could remove a patient's symptoms and even cure them by using hypnosis to **remove** a pathogenic fixed idea. Both experiments showed that fixed ideas, or, in a larger sense, the mind itself, can cause physical illness. Let's look at Janet's work.

Janet published a number of case studies of patients in which he used hypnosis to remove pathogenic fixed ideas from their mind. The following is a brief summary of one of those case studies in which he cured a patient named Marie.

In his treatment of Marie, Janet proved that an idea in the mind could cause both physical and mental symptoms. When he removed a specific fixed idea from Marie's mind, a whole cluster of her symptoms immediately disappeared, suggesting that the symptoms were caused by the fixed idea that Janet removed. Many of Marie's symptoms centered around her menstrual cycle. Here is a very brief portion of Janet's lengthy description of her symptoms:

> "At the time preceding her menstruations, Marie's character would change; she became gloomy and violent ... things went almost normal during the first day, but ... 20 hours after the beginning, the menstruation stopped suddenly and a great tremor would seize her whole body; then, a sharp pain ascended slowly from the abdomen to the throat, and a great hysterical crisis ensued. The attacks, although they were very violent, never lasted a long time, and had never resembled epileptoid tremors; instead, there was a very long and severe delirium."[20]

In the course of Marie's therapy, Janet thought it was relevant to find out more about her first period, which seems sensible given that

---

20 Gottschalk, S. (n.d.). How biographical treatments of Quimby and Eddy have influenced the development of New Thought and Christian Science. Retrieved from https://ppquimby-mbeddydebate.com/wp-content/uploads/2017/01/ppq-mbe-book-chapter-1.pdf

her symptoms were centered around her menstrual periods. He asked her several times to recount her memories of her first menstruation.

At first, and for many sessions afterward, she said she was simply unable to remember anything at all about it. This went on for a long time until Janet decided to hypnotize Marie. Under hypnosis, Marie recalled and described the whole difficult experience of her first menstruation: She had tried to stop that first period by dousing herself in ice-cold water because she was ashamed. She thought something bad was happening, and she tried to stop it by submersing herself in freezing water.

As a result, at the time of that first period, she had suffered almost all the same symptoms she was now having every time she menstruated. In other words, Marie was reliving the experience of that first traumatic menstruation every time she had a period now, later in her life.

When Marie recalled that memory of her first menstruation in hypnosis, Janet did an interesting thing. He transformed her memory. In the new memory of that first period, everything went well and she had a normal period. This entirely cured Marie of her symptoms! After that, her periods were always a normal experience for her.

In summary, Marie had a traumatic memory of her first menstrual period that was causing her to relive that trauma every time she had a period. When that memory was transformed into a positive memory, Marie stopped reliving the original trauma.

Case studies like this one were a further and different kind of proof that the mind can cause physical illness. Janet removed many of her symptoms by transforming a fixed idea in her mind, proving that the fixed idea—the original traumatic memory—was the cause of those symptoms.

Removing bacteria from the lung cures pneumonia. Removing a traumatic memory from the mind cures a case of PTSD.

Given that Charcôt's and Janet's work were part of a larger vein of clinical research going on in the second half of the 19th century, there are two crucial things to understand about this research:

1. It was moving towards the end of proving that fixed ideas are the cause of both physical and mental illness.
2. This discovery got lost in the excitement that surrounded the appearance of Sigmund Freud's ideas about sexuality.

Freud's theories about sexuality and the mind were first published in the 1890s. His theories went through several different stages, but all of them were grounded in the basic idea that sexual problems are the cause of mental illness. These theories landed in the midst of European society at the end of the 19th century, when sexuality and all talk of sexuality was rigorously repressed. In this setting, any mention of sex was exciting, and Freud's theory that repressing sexuality causes mental illness created a sensation.

As a result, Freud's theories about sexuality and the mind became a phenomenon, attracting an immense amount of attention. After some initial resistance, they became the accepted and dominant theory of the day. This meant that the up-and-coming theory that fixed ideas cause illness got lost in all the tumult and excitement surrounding Freud's revelations about sex.

However, the basic idea that the mind can cause physical illness did not die. It lived on in psychoanalytic theory, the name given to Freud's and his successors' body of work that describes how the mind works, and how the mind creates mental illness.

For about seven decades between 1910 and 1980, psychoanalytic theory was the foundation of the practice of just about all psychiatry. If you went to a doctor or hospital in those years to get help for a psychological problem or a mental illness, the doctors you would have seen were all believers, to one degree or another, in psychoanalysis. Those doctors would have seen and diagnosed your problems through the lens of psychoanalytic theory, and they would have treated you accordingly. They might have told you that you were having problems because you wanted to kill your father and make love with your mother, or that you were fixated at the oral stage of psychosexual development. And so forth.

Today, psychoanalysis is virtually a historical footnote, and very few psychiatrists follow the model.

The psychiatry of our day has been taken over by the biological model. After decades of believing Freud's theories that said that all mental illness is caused by sexual problems, the pendulum has swung all the way to the other side. We now believe that all mental problems and all mental illness are caused by biological disturbances of the brain and nervous system.

To give you an idea of the impact of the biological model of psychiatry, if you had an adolescent daughter who was acting out sexually, having sex with anyone and everyone in search of a sense of self-worth and love, psychiatry, as it is presently configured, would have your daughter take medicine to cure the problem. (Would you prefer this, or would you rather have her sit down and talk about life with a wise, good-hearted female therapist?)

During those seven decades when psychoanalysis was the be all and end all of psychiatry, it was still generally believed that the mind could cause physical illness. This type of disease—physical disease caused by the mind—was called psychosomatic illness, and the dominant theories of how the mind caused psychosomatic illness were psychoanalytic theories. In general, these theories held that psychodynamic conflicts, conflicts in the mind, cause psychosomatic illness.

The psychoanalytic theories were often flamboyant and far-fetched. For example, famous psychoanalyst Franz Alexander held that ulcers were caused by a patient's conflicted longing for love. Another influential psychoanalytic theory was that asthma is caused by a conflict between the patient and a domineering and overprotective parent. At the time, people believed these theories, but, in most quarters, they are simply misguided history now.

In the end, the psychoanalytic theories of psychosomatic illness faded and lost their influence for three basic reasons: (1) People realized, after a while, that they were just too far-fetched to believe; (2) they didn't work—therapy based on these theories didn't really help anyone; and

(3) with the ascendance of biological psychiatry, they were replaced by the biological theories of stress, which seemed more "scientific," as many psychiatrists were, in general, desperate to find more scientific explanations for the causes of both mental and psychosomatic illness.

In much the same fashion, the psychoanalytic period of psychiatry ended for a number of similar reasons: (1) Psychoanalysis did not work that well and was especially poor at treating the psychoses—for example, schizophrenia and manic depression; (2) it wasn't for everyone as it was a very intellectual form of therapy requiring the patient to be in therapy for years and even decades; and (3) with the change in health policy at the end of the century, there was a need to give increasing numbers of people therapy for mental problems. There simply wasn't enough time and money to pay for years of psychoanalysis for everyone—not to mention the fact that it didn't seem to work all that well. Insurance companies would simply not pay for it.

So psychoanalysis fell by the wayside, and the pendulum swung to the other extreme. Biological psychiatry rose to the fore, and that's why just about everyone who goes to see a psychiatrist gets medicine now instead of psychotherapy.

With the passing of psychoanalysis, and the ascendance of biological psychiatry, the mind was demoted within the field of psychiatry. It got left in the dust! We simply stopped thinking that the mind is the cause of either psychological or bodily illness. We began to believe that all mental illness is caused by biological lesions.

This era of biological psychiatry has given us a general theory of how extremely stressful situations—for example, the death of a spouse, a divorce, a demeaning and demanding boss at work, taking out a large mortgage that you are not sure you can repay—and even everyday stresses can cause physical illness.

This theory explains the genesis of physical stress by describing the physiological mechanisms by which stressful situations create stress within the body. To be more precise, it describes how the brain, pituitary gland, and adrenal gland work together to marshal the body's resources so that it can deal with and fight off the outer and inner stressors that occur in our lives.

This sequence of actions that the brain, pituitary gland, and adrenal gland take to adapt to and fight off stress is called the general adaptation syndrome (GAS), which prepares the body to fight off an external stress by giving it more energy using three different hormones secreted by the adrenal gland: (1) cortisol, which gives the body more energy by increasing the amount of glucose in the body (glucose is the fuel that energizes much of what happens in the body); (2) adrenalin; and (3) noradrenalin, which increase your heart rate and blood pressure, which in turn increases your energy level and gets you ready for action.

Although this GAS theory does an excellent job of explaining how stressful situations create stress in the body, it does not explain how the emotions cause specific, chronic, physical illness. Mainstream medicine simply does not know how to diagnose or treat illnesses—including chronic ones—caused by the emotions because modern medicine is wedded to the idea that biological lesions cause all illness. This theory is actually the foundation of modern medicine, and in many respects it is a very good theory.

Called the anatomo-clinical paradigm, this theory tells us, for example, that the biological lesion that defines and that is pneumonia is a portion of infected lung tissue. In much the same way, this theory also tells us that a stroke is caused by one of two different lesions: either an accumulation of fat— an atherosclerotic plaque—that reduces blood flow in an artery that takes blood to the brain, or the rupture of an artery that takes blood to the brain because the artery is either too weak or your blood pressure is too high.

Medicine, as it is now practiced, is entirely based on the idea that specific biological lesions cause specific diseases—even illnesses of the mind. This theory is both the strength and weakness of modern medicine.

The anatomo-clinical paradigm is a strength when your disease really is caused by a biological lesion. For example, if you go to the emergency room with a stroke, your doctors will know (once they have diagnosed that you have had a stroke) to look right away for one of the two lesions than can cause a stroke—either a blocked or ruptured artery. They know that they have to look for the lesion that has caused the stroke. This is how diagnosis works in modern medicine. Find the lesion causing the illness.

Once they find the lesion, your doctor's next step will be to treat that lesion. So, if you have an illness caused by a biological lesion (as with a stroke), the anatomo-clinical paradigm is very helpful. However, it is almost useless if you have a disease caused by the mind, which encompasses approximately 80 percent of all human illness. (Most doctors are in general agreement with this figure.) That is a lot of our illness! This means that we desperately need to understand both how emotions cause illness and how to cure those illnesses.

Please take this knowledge to heart. The mind causes the greater proportion of our illness! This means that if you have an illness caused by your emotions and ideas, there is nothing to be ashamed of. This is simply the way that things work. We all get into situations in our lives that generate thoughts and emotions that cause illness to develop in our bodies. This is an insight I've taken to heart. In contrast to mainstream medicine, I've developed a full repertoire of methods for both diagnosing and treating illnesses caused by the mind in general, and emotions in particular. I use proven methods both to determine when an emotion or idea is stuck in the body and causing illness and to clear those pathogenic emotions and ideas from the body. My methods cure the illnesses the mind creates. I have been studying and successfully treating diseases caused by the mind for more than 10 years now.

The next question to consider is an important one, and it touches upon all our lives: How do you know whether an illness you have is being caused by your mind? How do you know if you need the help of a doctor—a doctor like me—who has the ability to diagnose and cure physical illnesses caused by the mind?

There are two basic answers to this question:

1. If your doctor tells you that you have an illness for which the cause is not known, then it is entirely possible that your illness is being caused by an emotion or emotions that have gotten stuck in your body.
2. If your doctor tells you that you have a chronic disease that can be treated but not cured, it is probably an illness being caused by emotions.

The common thread in both situations is your doctor telling you that they do not know the cause of your illness. Allow me to explain!

Whenever you go to see your doctor for an illness or a symptom of some kind, the first thing that your doctor is going to do is to try to diagnose your problem by looking for the biological lesion causing your illness. For example, if you go to your doctor with a sore throat, swollen glands, and a fever, they will look to see if you have a strep infection of your throat, a common cause of this group of symptoms. In other words, strep throat is a biological lesion that can cause these symptoms, so your doctor will likely look for this by scanning your throat with a flashlight and tongue depressor and taking a culture of your throat to see if there are any streptococcus bacteria living there.

If your doctor sees that your throat is red, and that there is white pus-like fluid sitting on the surface of your throat, this will suggest to your doctor that you have a strep infection. If your culture is positive—if strep bacteria are found in your culture plate—you definitely have strep throat.

Here is another example. If you are an elderly man, and you come into an emergency room with pressing pain in the middle of your chest and shortness of breath, your doctor's first thought will be that you might be having a heart attack, a *myocardial infarct*, which is a piece of heart tissue that is dead or dying because it is not getting sufficient blood flow and oxygen. This is the biological lesion that causes the symptoms of a heart attack, and your doctor will almost certainly search for this lesion.

Your doctor will draw your blood for testing and measure the electrical activity in your heart by doing a test called an electrocardiogram. If certain enzymes show up in your blood, and if the electrical activity in your heart is abnormal in a characteristic way, your doctor will know that you have the biological lesion that we call a myocardial infarct. Again, this is the basic modus operandi of medicine.

But what happens if you go to the doctor with a problem, and your doctor is unable to find a cause—a biological lesion—for your illness? It could mean one of three different things:

1. It might mean that you don't really have a physical illness. Doctors are trained to recognize the existence of a finite number of specific symptoms, such as chest pain, a headache, shortness of breath after climbing two flights of stairs, or a burning pain on urination.

    If you go to your doctor with a symptom that no one has ever heard of, your doctor will probably tell you that you are not really sick. This is the kind of situation in which an unskillful doctor might tell you that "it is all in your head," that your mind is creating the symptom you are experiencing, not your body.

2. It might mean that you have a known illness, but, for some reason, your doctor is not able to diagnose it. This happens all the time in medicine. A patient goes to a doctor with a genuine physical illness, but their doctor is unable to figure out what the illness is. This can happen for a number of reasons that include:

    a. **The symptoms you have are an unusual presentation for the disease you have**. For example, if you are having a heart attack and the only symptom you have is heartburn. Usually a heart attack presents with the symptoms of chest pain and shortness of breath. So if your only symptom is heartburn, it is easy to imagine that your doctor might miss the diagnosis of heart attack.

    **b. The illness you have is a very rare illness, or perhaps a previously unknown illness.** This can really happen. For example, AIDS was an entirely new and unknown illness when patients with AIDS first started showing up to see doctors in the late 1970s. Before that time, AIDS did not exist, making it impossible for doctors to diagnose the first patients who had what we now call AIDS.

    **c. Your doctor is incompetent.**

3. The third basic possibility is that you have a known chronic disease for which the cause is unknown. In this case, your doctor will be able to diagnose and even treat your illness, but they will not be able to cure it by removing its cause.

For example, if you have a burning pain in your upper abdomen because you have too much acid in your stomach—called heartburn in television commercials and dyspepsia by medicine—your doctor will easily diagnose you with dyspepsia, but they will not be able to cure it. Most cases of dyspepsia are chronic, and the greater likelihood is that you will have to take medicine to relieve your heartburn for the rest of your life. Moreover, you will have to take even more of your medicine whenever you drink a lot of alcohol or coffee.

If the medicine you take for heartburn is not curing you, then what is it doing? It disrupts the pathogenesis of your heartburn and makes you feel better. In fact, most medicines doctors give their patients for chronic diseases interfere with the pathogenesis of those diseases in one way or another.

To understand what this means, let's take another look at the difference between the cause of a disease and its pathogenesis. The cause of a disease is the single variable or variables that set the disease in motion. Bacteria cause pneumonia. A genetic defect causes Down syndrome, and so forth. The pathogenesis of an illness is the cluster of physiological processes set in motion by the cause that create the disease and its symptoms.

The following diagram illustrates the relationship between the cause of a disease, its pathogenesis, and the disease itself:

*Cause – – > Pathogenesis – – > Disease*

*Fig. 1: The relationship between the cause of a disease, its pathogenesis, and the disease itself*

To understand this diagram better, let's look at another example. Cigarette smoking causes lung cancer. When you smoke, tar and nicotine get deposited on the surface of your bronchi, the pipes that bring air to your lungs. The tar and nicotine set in motion a series of chemical processes in your bronchi that create the lung cancer. Smoking is the cause of lung cancer, and the chemical processes that it generates to cause the growth of the lung cancer are its pathogenesis.

Here is another example. The tuberculosis bacterium is the cause of tuberculosis. The presence of tuberculosis bacteria in your body sets off a whole panoply of chronic inflammatory processes that create the lesions of tuberculosis and its symptoms. These inflammatory processes are the pathogenetic processes of tuberculosis.

The treatments we give patients for chronic diseases disrupt the pathogenesis of the symptoms of the disease.

For instance, in the case of heartburn, or dyspepsia, we know a great deal about the pathogenetic processes that create heartburn, but we do not know what gets those processes going in the first place. We know that stomach acid is produced by a specific type of cell in the lining of the stomach called a **parietal cell**, and we know the details of how the parietal cell creates that acid and injects it into the inner cavity of the stomach.

These processes by which the parietal cell produces acid are all part of the pathogenesis of heartburn because heartburn is generated by the excess production of acid in the stomach. If we can slow down the production of acid, we can relieve the symptom of heartburn, and this is exactly what we do. We have developed several different medications—called proton pump inhibitors—that disrupt the process by which the parietal cells produce acid in the stomach.

This is not, however, the only method that medicine has developed to disrupt the pathogenesis of dyspepsia. We have a second means that works really well.

A group of receptors in the stomach, called **histamine$_2$ receptors**, regulate how much acid gets produced and secreted into the stomach. A histamine$_2$ receptor is a molecule found on the surface of the parietal cells in the stomach. When a histamine molecule lands on and binds to a histamine$_2$ receptor, it causes the parietal cell to produce more acid in the stomach.

There is a group of medications called **histamine$_2$ antagonists** that bind to the histamine$_2$ receptor and block histamine from binding to the histamine$_2$ receptor. By blocking the histamine, these medicines decrease the amount of acid that the parietal cells secrete into the stomach. This then is our second means of blocking the pathogenesis of heartburn.

This also answers our original question: Why do patients with dyspepsia get better if the medicine we give them does not cure them? Because the medications we give patients for dyspepsia disrupt the pathogenesis of the symptom of heartburn.

This is also a general principle. Many medications that we use to treat patients with chronic diseases make them feel better by disrupting the pathogenesis of their illness. Those medications can provide truly effective symptomatic treatment for a chronic illness.

They can prevent heartburn by decreasing stomach acid production. They can restore normal breathing for a patient with asthma by dilating the patient's bronchial tubes. They can reduce or even eliminate chronic back pain by reducing the inflammation in your backbones.

These medications that disrupt the pathogenesis of a disease can do a lot of good. Dyspepsia, for example, used to be a debilitating disease that could require surgery to remove the stomach or even kill people. Now, more often than not, it's a disease that's easily managed.

There are many other illnesses for which we can now do a reasonably good job of treating by disrupting the pathogenesis of their symptoms, including asthma, arthritis, autoimmune diseases, depression, diabetes, and many more.

There is much to be grateful for. Countless patients are still alive and leading high quality lives because they received medications that disrupt the pathogenesis of the symptoms of their illness.

Yet, at the same time, we can and should do better. We are not curing these illnesses. We are simply making them more tolerable by giving patients symptomatic treatment. If we understood how emotions cause chronic illness, we could cure them.

There is one more problem. We are also padding the coffers of the pharmaceutical industry, sometimes for medications that don't do any good. We will be talking about this large problem at length in the next chapter by discussing a case study that involves cholesterol, heart attacks, strokes, and the pharmaceutical industry. We could just as easily discuss the opioid crisis.

# CHAPTER 3

# CHOLESTEROL, OPIODS, AND THE TRUTH

*"The pharmaceutical industry isn't the only place where there's waste and inefficiency and profiteering. That happens in much of the rest of the health care industry."*

— Marcia Angell, former editor,
*New England Journal of Medicine*

Likely you've already heard of statins, a family of medications used to lower the level of cholesterol in your blood. Doctors all over the world routinely prescribe statins for the purpose of preventing heart attacks and strokes. The first statin was approved for clinical use in 1987, and they became part of the American way of life in the 1990s.[21] Someone in your family is probably taking a statin right now.

Statins prevent heart attacks and strokes by thwarting the growth of fatty deposits on the inside of your arteries. These deposits (called *atherosclerosis*, which we mentioned earlier in the book) cause heart attacks and strokes by clogging, narrowing, and blocking your arteries. The important thing to know about statins is that they don't cure atherosclerosis. They don't stop the growth of its fatty deposits once

---

21 https://jamanetwork.com/journals/jamacardiology/fullarticle/2583424

and for all. At best, they slow it down. In addition, although statins do reduce the rate of heart attacks and strokes somewhat, it is only a tiny bit. Nonetheless, statins have, as a group, become the largest-selling medications in the world.

This is a classic example of how the modern pharmaceutical industry works. The industry makes massive amounts of money manufacturing drugs that treat chronic diseases without curing them, although these drugs often help a patient feel better. This is, remember, why a disease becomes chronic—it can't be cured. It remains with a person for as long as they live, meaning that patient has to take their medications for the rest of their lives—if they can afford to. There's a lot of money to be made off medications that have to be taken forever.

Statins aren't the only medication meant to be taken for the duration of a person's life, nor are they the only medication that reap massive profits while failing to cure the disease for which they are being used. The medications we take for high blood pressure, rheumatoid arthritis, multiple sclerosis, and ulcers all have to be taken for the rest of our lives, to name just a few.

Since I began writing this book, COVID-19 has swept across the planet and altered the pharmaceutical model in ways that even I could not have predicted. The most current profit models are staggering and have all but knocked the majority of the medications in 2018 from the top of this list.[22] With that said, we will continue to take a look at the list of the 10 most profitable drugs by sales in 2018 in the United States. Every single medication on that list is used to treat one chronic disease or another—treat it, but not cure it. The 10th-top-selling medication—an anticoagulant used to treat coronary artery disease—brought in **$6.5 billion** in 2018.[23] The leading medication—a medication used to treat chronic autoimmune diseases—raked in **$19.9 billion**—without curing the diseases it treats.

---

[22] https://www.drugdiscoverytrends.com/50-of-2022s-best-selling-pharmaceuticals/
[23] https://www.consumerreports.org/consumerist/what-are-the-10-biggest-money-making-prescription-drugs-and-what-do-they-treat/

Needless to say, statins are very big business. Lipitor, the first blockbuster statin, totaled sales of a mere **$94 billion** between 1992 and 2017.[24] That's about one eighth of the Pentagon's budget for 2020.

Americans spent a paltry $16.9 billion on statins in 2012 alone. In that year, more than $5 billion was spent on a single statin named Crestor, the third-best-selling medication in the USA that year.

A market of this size yields profits that the pharmaceutical industry is in no rush to lose. Indeed, the industry has gone to great scheming lengths to hold onto this market even though a growing body of scientific evidence shows that statins aren't all that effective.

Statins don't prevent that many heart attacks or strokes, and one impeccable study showed that taking a statin for several years prolonged a patient's life for a grand total of **four whole days**. In addition, a bundle of evidence has established that statins have an excessive number of side effects, some of which are monstrous.

To understand how a medication racks up massive profits even though it's not all that effective, let's take a look at the story of how statins came to be such a profitable, widely used drug.

After a century of intense research on atherosclerosis, medicine convinced itself that lowering the amount of cholesterol in the blood would prevent heart attacks and strokes. The basic idea was that if you could reduce the amount of cholesterol in a person's blood, it would slow down the rate at which cholesterol is deposited in the arteries, and this, in turn, would prevent heart attacks and strokes. Given that cholesterol is the principal component of the fatty deposits created by atherosclerosis in our arteries, this seemed reasonable. So scientists began to search for medications that would decrease the amount of cholesterol in the blood. Statins were what they found.

As matters stand now, if there is any truism thought to be beyond question by modern medicine, it's the theory that reducing cholesterol in the blood will reduce the rate of coronary artery disease, heart attacks,

---

24 https://www.fiercepharma.com/pharma/from-old-behemoth-lipitor-to-new-king-humira-u-s-best-selling-drugs-over-25-years

and strokes. This idea has had vast consequences. It led to the now mainstream practice of giving statins to large swathes of our population to keep them from having heart attacks. This was the right thing to do, wasn't it?

Not so fast.

As we said earlier, atherosclerosis is a process in which cholesterol is deposited on the inner wall of arteries. When cholesterol builds up in an artery, it gets hard and is called plaque—atherosclerotic plaque.

Healthy arteries are soft, flexible tubes, but when cholesterol builds up in an artery and forms plaque, the artery hardens and becomes stiff. The problem with cholesterol plaque is that when it takes up residence in the coronary artery—the artery that feeds the heart—it narrows the artery, and, as a result, less blood gets to the heart. When there isn't enough blood getting through to the heart, the heart muscle can get injured and even die. This is one of two mechanisms by which atherosclerosis can cause heart disease.

The second mechanism is this: If a cholesterol plaque gets large enough, it can break up into fragments. If this happens, a fragment can get stuck in the coronary artery and completely block blood flow to the heart. This is the cause of the massive heart attacks that kill a person on the spot.

In much the same way, if cholesterol deposits build up in one of the arteries that bring blood to the brain, it can cause a stroke. The mechanisms by which cholesterol plaques cause strokes are exactly the same as they are in heart attacks: Plaque can clog an artery and slow down blood flow to the brain, or a piece of plaque can break off and entirely stop blood flow to the portion of the brain normally fed by that artery.

In the scientific world right now, thanks to evidence gathered over a long period of time, there is no doubt that the accumulation of cholesterol in arteries causes heart attacks. The very first step in the sequence of discoveries that led to this realization was the act of simply seeing cholesterol plaque in an artery.

The great artist Leonardo da Vinci (1452–1519), who tirelessly studied human anatomy to improve his art, found atherosclerosis in one of his dissections, and he may have been the first to describe it.[25] Just simply seeing the stuff was the beginning of five centuries of scientific discovery that eventually led to the realization that atherosclerosis causes heart attacks.

The next record we have of someone seeing atherosclerosis came three centuries later. In 1799, British physician Caleb Hillier Parry found a gritty, fatty substance in the coronary arteries of sheep.[26] Sheep? Parry had been doing experiments on sheep to try to discover the cause of angina pectoris—the pressing chest pain that is the principal symptom of heart attacks in human beings.

After he discovered this gritty stuff in the coronary artery of his sheep, Parry became the first scientist to suggest that this clogging of the coronary artery might be the cause of heart disease. This was a little more than 200 years ago.

By the beginning of the 19th century, two people—da Vinci and Parry—had observed and recorded the existence of the stuff we now call atherosclerosis. In addition, Parry had even floated the theory that when this stuff blocks the coronary artery, it might cause heart disease. This all seems obvious to us now, but back then, these were large steps forward.

In 1768, before Parry, an English doctor named William Heberden was the first to actually describe angina pectoris.[27] Heberden described it as a squeezing, pressing pain in the chest that comes on when a person is in the midst of physical exertion of some kind—walking, running, or rowing a boat, for example.

At more or less the same time, Edward Jenner (the same Edward Jenner who discovered the smallpox vaccine) was the first person to speculate that there might be a connection between that pressing chest pain and clogged coronary arteries. He had done an autopsy on a physi-

---

25 https://www.britannica.com/biography/Leonardo-da-Vinci
26 https://en.wikipedia.org/wiki/Caleb_Hillier_Parry
27 http://www.epi.umn.edu/cvdepi/essay/william-heberden-on-angina-pectoris-1772/

cian who died during an attack of angina, and he noticed that the man's coronary artery was virtually solid.

Then, in 1858, Rudolph Virchow (the father of the field of pathology who, as we saw earlier, discovered that diseases of the organs are actually diseases of the cells of organs) did a series of autopsies in which he found that accumulations of fat were often present in the walls of the arteries of people who died of heart attacks.[28] This finding lent further credence to the idea that a clogged coronary artery could cause both chest pain and sudden death from a heart attack.

Another 20 years later, two German scientists—Carl Weigert and Karl Huber—realized that this same fatty substance really could block the coronary artery and reduce the flow of blood to the heart.[29] They gave the name "atherosclerosis" to this fatty substance, and the name stuck. (The name is Greek in origin. "Athero" means "cheese" in Greek and "sclerosis" means "hardening." Atherosclerosis was described as the buildup of a cheesy material inside arteries that caused the arteries to harden and narrow.) Now medicine was beginning to conclude that the buildup of this cheesy substance in the coronary artery could cause chest pain and sudden death. The next step was to figure out exactly what this cheesy substance was.

In 1908, a Russian scientist did an experiment in which he was able to induce a buildup of atherosclerosis in the arteries of rabbits by feeding them nothing but egg yolks and milk—a high-fat diet.[30] On dissection, the rabbits all had massive deposits of this cheesy stuff inside their arteries, raising the possibility that the cheesy deposits contained fat. At this point in the history of science, a mere century ago, no one knew what was actually in these atherosclerotic deposits.

Then, two short years later, in 1910, German chemist Adolf Windaus made a major discovery.[31] He found that the cheese-like plaques that

---

28 https://www.aaas.org/rudolph-virchow-father-cellular-pathology
29 https://www.ncbi.nlm.nih.gov/pmc/articles/PMC10257777/
30 https://www.ncbi.nlm.nih.gov/pmc/articles/PMC1764970/
31 https://www.britannica.com/biography/Adolf-Windaus

caused atherosclerosis were full of cholesterol. This was a large step forward.

In 1913, two Russian scientists added yet more proof to the theory that the plaques were made of cholesterol.[32] Feeding a pure cholesterol diet to rabbits, they found that it produced both increased levels of cholesterol in the rabbit's blood and a massive amount of atherosclerosis in their aortas (the large artery that starts at the left ventricle and is the first artery to leave the heart).

Now medicine was beginning to understand three basic things about cholesterol and heart disease: (1) Cholesterol is the main component of the deposits of atherosclerosis; (2) high-cholesterol diets seem to cause atherosclerosis; and (3) cholesterol and atherosclerosis play a role in the causation of heart disease.

Norwegian doctor Carl Müller further confirmed these theories in 1939 when he discovered that whole families had excessively high levels of cholesterol in their blood.[33] It also turned out that members of these families were prone to having premature heart attacks. In other words, these families had a genetic defect that caused them to have astronomically elevated levels of cholesterol in their blood. More than that, the people of these families tended to have massive heart attacks in their 20s and 30s. These findings seemed to be strong evidence that high levels of blood cholesterol cause heart attacks.

Slowly, but surely, medicine was coming around to the realization that the accumulation of cholesterol in the coronary artery was the cause of heart attacks.

Strong, elegant confirmation of this theory came in the 1950s when American physiologist Ancel Keys conducted an incredible study of the health effects of diets in seven different countries.[34] Keys found two basic things: (1) People who consume diets high in cholesterol and saturated fats have a high level of cholesterol in their blood; and (2) a high level

---

32 https://www.ncbi.nlm.nih.gov/pmc/articles/PMC1764970/
33 https://sciencebasedmedicine.org/the-cholesterol-controversy/
34 https://www.sevencountriesstudy.com/about-the-study/investigators/ancel-keys/

of cholesterol in the blood increases the number of fatal heart attacks.[35] He came to these conclusions by studying several groups of people who consumed diets that contained dramatically different amounts of cholesterol and saturated fats.

For example, he studied a group of Finnish foresters who were in the habit of spreading butter on their cheese! In contrast, he also studied a group of Japanese fishermen who ate mostly fish, rice, and vegetables. When he measured the level of cholesterol in the Japanese fishermen's blood, he found that on average it was 165 milligrams. Not surprisingly, he found that the Finnish foresters' level was much higher at 270 milligrams. This difference in blood cholesterol was associated with a dramatic difference in the rate of heart attacks. The Finnish foresters suffered **13 times** more deaths from coronary heart disease than the Japanese fishermen.

Then, in 1961, the first results of the famous Framingham Study were published. Carried out by the National Heart Institute, this was a prospective study of 5,000 people who lived in Framingham, Massachusetts.[36] (A prospective study researches the causes of a disease by starting to study a group of people before they actually get the disease. The results of a prospective are thought to be especially reliable.) In Framingham, when the study began, none of the 5,000 people had ever had heart disease. The level of blood cholesterol was measured in each of the 5,000 subjects at the beginning of the study, and then the researchers followed them and recorded who did and didn't have heart attacks over the subsequent years of the study.[37]

The Framingham Study found that the individuals who had higher blood cholesterol levels at the beginning of the study were much more likely to have a heart attack than the subjects who had lower cholesterol levels at the beginning. With this study in hand, a tipping point was reached. Medical science was now convinced that an elevated level of

---

35 https://www.sevencountriesstudy.com/about-the-study/investigators/ancel-keys/
36 https://www.ncbi.nlm.nih.gov/pmc/articles/PMC4159698/
37 https://www.ncbi.nlm.nih.gov/pmc/articles/PMC4159698/

cholesterol in a person's blood was the primary cause of heart attacks.

This was an exciting discovery because it raised the possibility that reducing the level of cholesterol in a person's blood might prevent heart attacks. This seemed to be the path that medicine should pursue.

At the time, finding a way to prevent heart attacks was becoming an urgent matter and even a national priority in America because the rate of heart attacks had dramatically increased during the first half of the 20th century. It had become an epidemic.

At the end of the 19th century, heart attacks had been a relatively uncommon cause of death. In 1900, the top three causes of death in America were all infectious diseases—pneumonia, tuberculosis, and gastrointestinal infections.[38] They were the leading causes of death because antibiotics had yet to be discovered.

However, by the 1950s, heart disease was the most common cause of death in America, and it still is. Now, on average, more than 805,000 people have heart attacks in America every year, 164,000 of which are fatal.[39]

This graph of the incidence of heart disease in America shows how rapidly the rate of heart disease grew to become an epidemic in the first half of the 20th century:

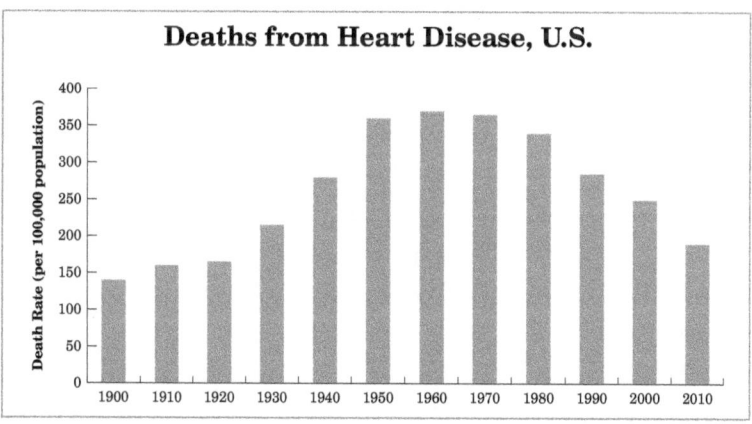

*Fig. 2: Incidence of heart disease in America in first half of 20th century*

---

38 https://www.cdc.gov/nchs/data/dvs/lead1900_98.pdf
39 https://www.verywellhealth.com/heart-attack-facts-and-statistics-5667421

Notice that the death rate for heart disease went up sharply in the first half of the century, and that it declined somewhat over the final four decades once we began to find ways to prevent and treat heart disease.

As this epidemic of heart attacks took hold and became a national problem, medicine turned its attention to finding a way to prevent them. The path ultimately chosen was to try to prevent heart attacks by blocking the synthesis of cholesterol in the body. The hope was that if a medicine could be found that would suppress the synthesis of cholesterol, this medicine could be used to decrease the level of cholesterol in a patient's blood. The expectation was that this would prevent heart attacks.

Given all the research done to date on cholesterol, this was a reasonable, obvious approach. However, the core of the theory upon which this approach was based—the idea that reducing the level of cholesterol in the blood would reduce the incidence of heart attacks—has turned out to be false. Even though high levels of cholesterol in the blood play a significant role in causing heart attacks, reducing cholesterol in the blood doesn't significantly reduce the rate of heart attacks.

Nobody anticipated this result, and it wasn't discovered until a lot of money had been invested in developing statins—medications now widely used by doctors all over the world to lower the level of cholesterol in the blood.

The starting point for the research that led to the discovery of medications that could reduce blood cholesterol was this: **We need cholesterol to survive**.

Cholesterol is a principal constituent of the membranes that surround every cell in our bodies. Without cholesterol, our cells wouldn't have proper membranes, and healthy life wouldn't be possible. We definitely need cholesterol.

The problem comes when there is too much cholesterol in the blood, which, as we've discussed, plays a role in causing atherosclerosis and heart attacks.

The cholesterol we have in our bodies comes from two different sources: the food we eat and cholesterol synthesis within the body. The liver manufactures most of our cholesterol then ships it out to the rest of the body. Given this, medicine had two basic options for lowering cholesterol in the blood: One was reducing the amount of cholesterol in a person's diet; the other was finding a way to block the synthesis of cholesterol in the liver. Mainstream medicine decided on the second option—finding a medication that could block the synthesis of cholesterol.

Why did medicine take this approach instead of focusing on diet? For one, this is what modern medicine does. When it comes to treating chronic diseases, medicine likes to tinker around with the molecules that play a role in the development of those diseases. It does this with high blood pressure, rheumatoid arthritis, ulcerative colitis, and all the rest.

Secondly, your doctor might tell you to cut down on certain foods and eat better, but, in general, mainstream medicine doesn't really believe that low-cholesterol diets prevent heart attacks. Consider this revealing passage from a paper written by David G. Nathan of Harvard Medical School:

> "Although the excessive fat, simple starch, and sugar content of the American diet ... certainly contribute to high blood cholesterol, alteration of diet is an inefficient approach to the problem. First, only zealots stick to diets; most fall off the pledge. The cheapness of salt, sugar, and fat, the power of advertising, and the third-rate health education that has been thrust on many Americans have combined to produce a horribly fed public, particularly among the less educated and poor."

In general, modern medicine does not pay that much attention to nutrition. Doctors simply don't learn a great deal about nutrition in medical school. Dr. Vyner received just a one-hour lecture on nutrition as part of his physiology course in his entire four years in medical school.

Nonetheless, it might be possible to prevent heart attacks by putting people on a proper diet. Several good studies have shown that eating a Mediterranean diet really does reduce the incidence of heart attacks—

without sacrificing the joy of eating. After all, Italians seem to know what they're doing in the kitchen.

All in all, medicine is much more interested in giving medications to its patients than it is in recommending a change in nutrition or lifestyle that will genuinely prevent heart attacks. At this point in medical history, mainstream medicine is fixated on finding and prescribing medicines that will disrupt the biochemical reactions that bring a disease to life.

This is exactly what we have done with the problem of heart attacks. We set out to find a way to prevent heart attacks by suppressing the synthesis of cholesterol. Even though this approach made sense at the time, it didn't give us the ability to seriously reduce the number of heart attacks. Here's how it all unfolded.

Finding the solution to the problem of how to inhibit cholesterol synthesis—which involved an immense amount of sophisticated biochemical research—led to two Nobel Prizes. German scientists Konrad Bloch and Feodor Lynen won one in 1964 for playing a crucial role in mapping out the sequence of chemical reactions that leads to the synthesis of cholesterol.[40]

Along the way, they found the enzyme HMG-CoA reductase, which controls the rate of cholesterol synthesis. With this discovery, it became clear that the way to reduce the amount of cholesterol in the blood was to inhibit this enzyme. If a medication could be developed that would keep that enzyme from doing its job, this would suppress the synthesis of cholesterol and reduce the amount of cholesterol in the blood.

The second Nobel Prize went to American doctors Joseph Goldstein and Michael Brown of the University of Texas Southwestern Medical Center in Dallas. They discovered that if you suppress the synthesis of cholesterol in the body's cells, the cells will make up for the lost cholesterol by importing cholesterol into themselves from the bloodstream that feeds them.[41] This seemed perfect.

This finding meant that if science could find a medication that would

---

40 https://en.wikipedia.org/wiki/Feodor_Lynen
41 https://en.wikipedia.org/wiki/Joseph_L._Goldstein

block the action of HMG-CoA reductase, it would block the synthesis of cholesterol in the liver and reduce the level of cholesterol in the blood, preventing heart attacks.

In 1976, Japanese scientist Akira Endo discovered a molecule that had the ability to inhibit HMG-CoA reductase. He named this molecule compactin, and it was the first statin. Science would go on to discover and bring to market several more statins in the years to come.[42]

The discovery of compactin gave medicine exactly what it had been looking for: a means of disrupting the development of atherosclerosis and preventing heart attacks by reducing the amount of cholesterol in the blood. This is a typical strategy that modern medicine uses to treat chronic illnesses.

As matters stand now, medicine merely tries to retard the development of chronic diseases, and it seems to be stuck in its ways. It does not appear to have either the necessary perspective or the wisdom to cure chronic diseases, which plays right into the hands of the pharmaceutical industry. The industry is more than willing to supply medications that have to be taken forever—and rake in the profits.

Statins are a prime example of this limited approach to treating chronic illnesses. Nonetheless, statins have become a major market worldwide. Everyone—both doctors and patients—wants to prevent heart attacks and strokes, and the pharmaceutical industry has played into this desire by using rigged studies and dishonest advertising to convince everyone that statins can give them the ability to prevent heart attacks and strokes.

In 1987, the United States Food and Drug Administration (FDA) approved the first statin, Mevacor, for use by human beings.[43] At the time, there was no scientific evidence to show that Mevacor could prevent heart attacks or prolong life. Mevacor was approved solely on the strength of one study that showed that it could reduce the levels of cholesterol in the blood. For seven years, doctors prescribed statins without possessing

---

42 https://www.ncbi.nlm.nih.gov/pmc/articles/PMC4525717/
43 https://www.news-medical.net/health/Statin-History.aspx

any proof that they could prevent heart attacks.

The first study to show that statins could prevent heart attacks and prolong life was published in 1994. Sponsored by drug manufacturer Merck, it was called the Scandinavian Simvastatin Survival Study. It evaluated the effectiveness of a statin called simvastatin, which just happened to be a Merck product.

The study purported to show that simvastatin: (1) reduced blood cholesterol levels; (2) reduced the incidence of heart attacks; and (3) prolonged life. These very hopeful findings excited the medical world.

But notice that this study was bankrolled by Merck—the very company that manufactured simvastatin. You don't need a medical degree to understand that this arrangement might corrupt the findings of a study. Common sense alone tells you that if a drug study is funded by the company that makes it, this just might lead to biased results in favor of their drug. Nonetheless, it was thought to be a landmark study at the time.

Prior to the 1980s, the federal government funded the bulk of the medical research done in America, but the Reagan administration slashed research funding because President Reagan and his fellow Republicans believed in small government.

At first glance this might seem like a harmless move, but the drug companies rushed in to fill the void. They began to fund much of the research being done on their products. As a result, drug manufacturers have sponsored and funded the majority of the research studies ever done on the effectiveness of the statins they produce and market.

Of course, this isn't a good idea. Scientific studies have clearly shown that when corporations fund the research into their own medications, it produces biased results. For example, scientists at the University of California at San Francisco School of Medicine—one of our best medical schools—did a study that found that when a company funded research on its own medication, the research results were more likely to favor their drug.

This happens because the drug companies can manipulate the findings of their studies. The companies can and do use well-known methods to rig their statistics to get the results that they want, and this is exactly what happened with many of the studies claiming that statins are powerful preventers of heart attacks.

We're going to discuss one of the methods the drug companies used to distort their findings in a moment.

The Scandinavian Study financed by Merck wasn't the only research to evaluate the preventive abilities of statins. It was just the first one. Since the completion of that first study, more than 20 others purport to show that statins prevent heart attacks and prolong life.

In 2005, a milestone paper was published in prestigious British journal *The Lancet* that reviewed and evaluated the results of 14 major studies that claimed to show that statins are effective. This review study was done by a collaborative group of scores of doctors from both England and Australia.

Review studies are often a helpful strategy in medical research. They usually happen after a number of independent studies have been completed on the same issue, and their purpose is to evaluate and analyze the results of all those prior studies to give medicine the ability to see the larger picture.

For example, a review of this type might analyze the results of 10 different studies to evaluate the merits of using a shunt for patients who have had heart attacks and whether they prolong life. Or another review might evaluate and analyze 12 studies that looked at whether a particular high blood pressure medication prevents strokes, and so forth.

*The Lancet* paper that evaluated the statin research reviewed and analyzed 14 studies to determine if statins really do decrease heart attacks and/or prolong life. More than 90,000 patients had been followed by all these studies—a massive number of subjects. The results of a review of this magnitude should have given medicine an accurate picture of whether statins are effective.

*The Lancet* paper claimed that the 14 studies established beyond any doubt that statins do reduce heart attacks and prolong life. They even quantified the benefits. They found that for every 40 milligrams of reduction in a patient's blood cholesterol, a person's risk of having a heart attack was reduced by 20 percent.

Here's an example of what that means. If you have a cholesterol level of 340 when you first visit your doctor, and if you then reduced your cholesterol to 300 by taking a statin, *The Lancet* paper claimed that you would then have a 20 percent less risk of having a heart attack in the remainder of your life. If you reduced your blood cholesterol another 40 milligrams to 260, you would have a 40 percent less risk of having a heart attack, and so on. That sounds pretty good at first glance.

However, if you take a closer look at the statistical methods the individual studies used, it is easy to see that they oversold the effectiveness of statins. Some of these studies misrepresented and distorted their findings to make it look as though statins are much more effective than they really are.

To see how these 14 studies manipulated their findings, let's take a closer look at one of them that was analyzed by the landmark paper of *The Lancet* so that we can see what it really found.

We're going to the Anglo-Scandinavian Cardiac Outcomes Trial–Lipid-Lowering Arm (ASCOT- LLA) study. This was done by a group of prestigious doctors at prestigious institutions, yet the statistics were rigged to make it seem like statins were far more effective than they actually were.

## THE ASCOT-LLA STUDY[44]

The findings of the ASCOT-LLA study have been promoted in advertisements aimed at both the general public and the medical profession. They claimed that the ASCOT-LLA study proved that statins have a robust ability to prevent heart attacks. This study was widely publicized, and the advertisements that trumpeted its findings were clearly designed to encourage patients to ask their doctors to give them statins.

The ASCOT-LLA study looked at 10,305 patients who already had heart problems. Half the patients were given a statin and half were

---

[44] https://www.acc.org/latest-in-cardiology/clinical-trials/2010/02/22/19/05/ascot--lipid-arm

given a placebo. The patients were then followed to see how many heart attacks they had. The results of this study were manipulated to make it seem as though the statins were much more effective than they were. To understand how the results of this study were brazenly manipulated, we have to look at a few statistics.

The statistics were presented in a way that made it appear as though the drug being tested was a miracle drug when it wasn't. Here are the results: Of the patients in the placebo group, 3 percent had a heart attack during the study, whereas 1.9 percent of the patients in the group that received the statin had a heart attack. In other words, 97 percent of the patients who didn't get the statin did not have a heart attack. That is almost everybody!

Of the patients who did get the statin, 98.1 percent did not have a heart attack. This is a negligible increase. Out of every 100 patients, one additional person did not have a heart attack.

What do you think? Is this small improvement worth all the expense and effort of taking a statin? Is it worth the well-known risk of developing one of the drug's side effects?

Regardless of how common sense might read these results, this study was ballyhooed and marketed as evidence of the fact that statins are lifesaving drugs we should all be taking.

Many physicians came to believe that this study established the worth of Lipitor, the drug evaluated by this study. They were undoubtedly moved to prescribe Lipitor because the study claimed that Lipitor reduced the risk of heart attacks by 36 percent! Where did they get this figure? After all, there was only a 1.1 percent increase in the number of heart attacks in the untreated subjects!

Here's how they got it. They divided 3 percent—the percentage of people who had heart attacks in the placebo group—by 1.1 percent. This figure of 1.1 percent was the decrease in the percent of patients who had heart attacks; it is 36 percent of 3 percent. This is a blatant misrepresentation of the data, and of course they knew what they were doing.

More than that, Pfizer, the manufacturer of Lipitor, advertised the results of this study far and wide, claiming that Lipitor reduced the risk of heart attack by 36 percent.

The pharmaceutical industry seems to know no shame. They misrepresented their data and used that misrepresentation to relentlessly market the statins. Ultimately, even the pharmaceutical industry's preferred statin studies don't prove that these drugs are that effective.

But there is more to this story: as of 2017, 44 scientific studies have shown that lowering blood cholesterol does not prolong a person's life.

Think about this for a moment. This is important. The whole rationale for giving a patient a statin has been the theory that lowering the level of cholesterol in a person's blood would prolong their life by reducing the likelihood that they would have a heart attack. If it were true that statins prevent heart attacks and prolong life, then it would make good sense to prescribe them.

However, the results from 44 studies now show that cholesterol-lowering medications don't do what they're supposed to do. Every single one of these 44 studies found that giving a patient a medication that reduces their blood cholesterol doesn't prolong their life, and almost all of them found that lowering cholesterol does not prevent heart attacks.

In other words, the entire premise upon which the quest to find cholesterol-lowering drugs was based appears to have been wrong. This is a crucial point. The basic strategy of reducing cholesterol does not work. It does not prolong life.

But this didn't stop the pharmaceutical industry from aggressively marketing statins.

A now famous, remarkable Danish study found that if a person took a statin for two to six years, their life expectancy would be extended by an average of a **mere four days**. Four days! Does anyone really think that four days is worth the expense and the side effects of taking a statin?

Speaking of side effects, the largest survey ever done of patients taking a statin found that 46 percent of them stopped taking their statin because they developed at least one of its side effects. The most common side effects of statins are severe muscle pain and weakness, and the onset of type 2 diabetes. Not surprisingly, the pharmaceutical industry has gone to great lengths to fund research that minimizes the frequency of these side effects.

In much the same way that the industry manipulated their statin studies to make it look as though they are miracle drugs that will bring about the end of heart disease in the 21$^{st}$ century—a published prediction made by Nobel Laureates Brown and Goldstein—the industry has also distorted statistics to bolster the case that statins do not cause many side effects.

But there is more! We have not yet exhausted the repertoire of dirty tricks that the pharmaceutical industry brought to the task of marketing statins.

A central element of their marketing strategy was to prevail upon esteemed medical organizations to issue treatment guidelines that would lead doctors to prescribe statins for more and more of their patients. They even dreamed, as one industry scientist joked, of "putting statins in the water supply."

The final method that the pharmaceutical industry used to promote the widespread use of statins was to put their own people on the committees that are in the business of issuing treatment guidelines for heart disease.

In America, many medical organizations issue treatment recommendations for the illnesses in which they specialize. This is a routine practice and is often done with good intentions. The idea is to standardize and improve medical care by giving direction and advice to doctors who don't know much about a particular disease because it is not their specialty.

For example, the American Diabetes Association makes recommendations for the treatment of diabetes. This is a good idea because the treatment of diabetes can be very complicated. In much the same way, the American Heart Association makes recommendations for the treatment and prevention of heart disease, and so forth.

However, when you look at the people who are on the medical councils making recommendations for the use of statins, it becomes apparent that these councils were taken over by the companies that manufacture statins. For example, the US National Cholesterol Education Program (NCEP) is a program of the National Institutes of Health (NIH). Its stated purpose is to reduce the amount of heart disease caused by hypercholesterolemia—high levels of cholesterol in the blood. *The NCEP is in the business of issuing guidelines for the use of statins to prevent heart disease.*

In 2004, for example, the NCEP created a set of treatment guidelines that dramatically increased the number of patients that would be given a statin, and they did it by changing the definition of high blood cholesterol[45]—they lowered the level of cholesterol considered to be high. As a result, many people who were thought to have a normal cholesterol level prior to 2004 were suddenly now said to have too much cholesterol in their blood. This meant that doctors all over the country would end up prescribing statins to millions more of their patients. It goes without saying that the pharmaceutical companies manufacturing statins would be making a great deal more money as a result.

It turned out that NCEP's guidelines were biased. **Eight out of nine members** of the 2004 NCEP guideline committee were on the payroll of companies that manufacture statins.[46] This was not an isolated occurrence.

In 2013, the United Kingdom's National Institute for Health and Care Excellence (NICE) issued guidelines that would have dramatically increased the number of patients taking statins.[47] Guess what? The NICE panel that made these recommendations had 12 members. Eight of those 12 members had financial ties to companies that manufacture the medications that lower blood cholesterol.

All in all, this is not a pretty picture. First, the corporations that

---

45 https://link.springer.com/chapter/10.1007/978-0-387-76606-5_2
46 https://www.proquest.com/docview/2067714051
47 https://www.proquest.com/docview/2067714051

manufacture statins have been sponsoring and controlling the bulk of the research done on statins. They have distorted the results of those studies and used those distorted findings to aggressively market their products and swell their profits to obscene proportions. They have also used statistical ploys to downplay the side effects of statins.

As if that were not enough, the pharmaceutical industry has also placed their own scientists on the medical councils responsible for issuing guidelines for doctors about how best to use statins to prevent heart disease. These recommendations are very important because they have a huge effect. Doctors generally have faith in the guidelines issued by these trusted organizations; as a result, they will prescribe more statins.

This is all happening in the face of the fact that a great deal of scientific evidence makes the case that reducing cholesterol levels does not prevent heart attacks or prolong life. In other words, this whole effort to focus on reducing blood cholesterol looks to have been a big mistake.

However, this does not mean that it will not be possible to prevent heart attacks. The medical world is beginning to look elsewhere and wake up, with a great deal of research beginning to show that insulin resistance is actually the cause of our heart attack epidemic.

Insulin is naturally present in our bodies, and, like cholesterol, we need it. It promotes the movement of sugar into our cells, which is important because sugar is a major source of energy for the cells. Insulin resistance is a condition in which the body's cells do not respond to insulin in the proper fashion; however, we can eliminate it without taking medications. A number of studies have shown that eating a Mediterranean-style diet will simultaneously lower insulin resistance and prevent heart attacks. However, there is not much profit to be made in prescribing dietary changes, and it won't win anyone a Nobel Prize.

Nonetheless, as more research is done, we believe the medical world will eventually see the light and change its approach to preventing heart attacks. We will start to focus on lowering insulin resistance to prevent heart attacks, and the emphasis will be on establishing healthy nutrition and making lifestyle changes.

We also believe that the scientists who did the original cholesterol and statin research meant well. They must have believed that they were working for the good of humanity. We want to think that they thought they were searching for a way to tamp down the epidemic of heart attacks that was—and still is—ravaging modern civilization. It's the plague of our day.

However, we can accuse the scientists of being shortsighted. They must not have considered the idea that patients' lifestyles and diets might be causing this epidemic. After all, this epidemic began in the first half of the 20$^{th}$ century. Something about modern life causes heart attacks.

Without realizing what they were doing, these scientists enabled the lifestyle that has created this heart attack epidemic: Many people thought they could eat anything they wanted if they just took their statins.

In the end, though, it is the pharmaceutical industry that has made a mammoth mess of the situation. They took the scientists' well-intended work and turned it into a huge ATM machine. The pharmaceutical industry has to be one of the most conniving, sneaky, underhanded, manipulative industries in existence and makes for a terrible bedmate for health care.

There are two morals to this story. First, mainstream medicine needs to change its approach to preventing heart attacks and strokes. Second, we must find a way to rein in the pharmaceutical industry. The marketing of statins is not the only example of corruption that has happened in this industry. Many times, the pharmaceutical industry has pursued profits at the expense of the health of the American people.

Another problem with the pharmaceutical industry is that it has a marked tendency to charge obscene amounts of money for its products—products that people need to be healthy and to save their lives.

Take the EpiPen, a device used to quickly inject epinephrine, also called adrenalin, into a patient who is having an anaphylactic reaction—a serious allergic response that is typically a reaction to nuts, seafood, or an insect bite. An anaphylactic reaction can kill a person within minutes by closing down their airway, and an injection of adrenalin will save their life.

Mylan, a pharmaceutical company in the Netherlands, acquired the right to market the EpiPen in 2007. In 2009, the cost of a two-pack of EpiPens was $106.50. Mylan then increased the price several times, and by May 2016, the price had grown to $608.61! At the time, the cost of the medication in the EpiPen—epinephrine—was 34 cents. In England, an EpiPen costs the equivalent of $69 and in France it is $100.

Then there is the infamous case of Daraprim, a medication used to treat parasitic diseases, and Martin Shkreli. Turing Pharmaceuticals, of which Shkreli was the CEO, acquired the marketing rights to Daraprim in 2015. Before that time, the price of a dose of Daraprim was $13.50. Shkreli immediately raised the price to $750 per dose. In India, which has an excellent pharmaceutical industry, the price of a single dose of Daraprim is 10 cents.

Another serious problem with the pharmaceutical industry is that it tends to hide the side effects of the drugs it manufactures. Consider the opioid crisis. Purdue Pharma and the Sackler family not only manufactured OxyContin; they manufactured the opioid crisis.

They sent drug reps to pressure doctors to prescribe OxyContin. They held conferences at fancy resorts and paid all the expenses for the doctors they invited to come hear their propaganda. They were even allowed to design pain control courses that trumpeted OxyContin to medical schools and doctors. They spent billions of dollars marketing this drug.

Worst of all, they lied about the most important detail. They knew that OxyContin was addictive. They knew that OxyContin was being crushed into powder so that it could be sold and snorted on the streets for its heroin-like high. But they lied and told the medical community that it was not addictive. We all now know better now, and Purdue Pharma has been fined billions of dollars—and counting—for their dishonesty.

Next, let's consider Johnson & Johnson's baby powder—a trusted, iconic American product if ever there was one. After all, they are "a family company." It turns out that this much used product was contaminated with asbestos, which causes several different types of cancer—including ovarian cancer and cancer of the pleura, the membrane that covers and protects the lungs.

J&J's baby powder became contaminated with asbestos because talc, a component of the product, is a mineral often found in deposits with asbestos. When you dig up the talc, you get asbestos as well. Johnson & Johnson knew about this asbestos contamination because they tested their product many times over the years; the tests found asbestos contamination—the first time in 1957![48] They found it again in the late 1960s.

Between 1972 and 1975, J&J hired three different labs to test their talc to see if it contained asbestos.[49] All three labs found asbestos, but J&J failed to tell the FDA about these tests. In its public statements, over and over again, J&J stated that its baby powder was absolutely free of asbestos. They even hired a consultant geologist who claimed at trials that the asbestos was not asbestos. And, of course, they kept selling their baby powder.

In essence, J&J deceived the public to maintain and expand their profits, and now they are being punished for it. In 2018, J&J was ordered to pay $4.7 billion in damages to 22 women who claimed that their products caused them to develop ovarian cancer. As matters stand now, there are more than 14,000 claims for cases of ovarian and pleural cancer. Unfortunately, as of the release of this book, J&J are still successfully occupying the courts in order to avoid a settlement.

Finally, there is the story of Vioxx, a nonsteroidal anti-inflammatory medication developed to treat the most common type of arthritis called osteoarthritis.

Vioxx was used to reduce pain and restore mobility to inflamed joints. In its first five years it was a wildly popular drug. In its short six years on the market, it brought in $11 billion for Merck, its manufacturer.

---

48 https://www.businessinsider.com/
johnson-and-johnson-knew-for-decades-baby-powder-contained-asbestos-2018-12

49 https://www.nbcnews.com/health/health-news/
johnson-johnson-knew-decades-asbestos-lurked-its-baby-powder-n948016

There was one small problem with Vioxx, however. It causes heart attacks.

Vioxx was sold on the American market for only six years, from 1999 to 2005. During this short period of time, the US Food and Drug Administration's office of drug safety has estimated that between 88,000 and 139,000 people (in the United States) suffered a heart attack or stroke as a result of taking Vioxx.[50] That is a lot of people, and it was also a serious mistake that could have been avoided.

It happened because Merck hid and manipulated the results of the research that showed that Vioxx would cause heart attacks and strokes.

Merck completed an in-house study in 1996 that showed that taking Vioxx markedly increases the risk of developing blood clots that cause heart attacks and strokes.[51] In 1998, Merck applied to the FDA for approval to sell Vioxx, failing to mention these studies in their application! Furthermore, they manipulated the data from the studies they did submit to the FDA to make it look as though Vioxx does not cause heart attacks.[52] The FDA approved Vioxx for sale in 1999.

Then, once Vioxx was on the market, Merck did further studies that found that taking Vioxx does increase the risk of heart attacks, but they manipulated the data, hid the risk, and continued to sell the drug anyway. Now Merck continues to market Vioxx in more than 80 countries around the world.

Clearly, the pharmaceutical industry has a tendency to allow profits to become more important than the health of its customers. The time has come to find a way to make certain that corporate profits cease to dictate the kind of medications that our doctors give us.

---

50 https://www.npr.org/2007/11/10/5470430/timeline-the-rise-and-fall-of-vioxx
51 https://www.ucsusa.org/resources/merck-manipulated-science-about-drug-vioxx
52 https://www.ucsusa.org/resources/merck-manipulated-science-about-drug-vioxx

# CHAPTER 4

# THE OUTLANDISH COST OF MEDICAL CARE IN AMERICA

*"Of all the forms of inequality, injustice in health is the most shocking and the most inhuman."*

—Dr. Martin Luther King Jr.

Everyone agrees. The cost of medical care in the United States is outrageously high. We pay far more for our health care than any other country in the world.

I see the problem with the cost of medical care in America as two-dimensional: It's not only too expensive, but the quality of medical care we get for our hard-earned money is sub-par. It's nowhere near the best in the world. The data backs this up.

First, let's look at the cost. Several different organizations regularly assess and compare the cost of health care worldwide. Although they come up with slightly different figures, one thing is always the same. The per capita cost of health care in America is far higher than the cost of medical care in any other country in the world.

The Organization for Economic Cooperation and Development (OECD) collects the most respected data on health care expenditures in the world. They found that the average American paid $12,914 for health care in 2021, the highest in the world.[53] The second-highest country was Germany where the per capita expenditure was $7,383.[54] We pay 40 percent more for our health care than the next highest country!

The disparity is even worse when you look at the average for all the OECD countries, which in 2021 was only $4,986.[55] That is 38 percent of what we pay, and, remember, the 38 countries in the OECD are all developed countries with high income economies.

Another way to evaluate a country's health care expenditures is to measure how much it spends on health care as a portion of its gross domestic product (GDP). In 2021, the United States spent 17.8 percent of its GDP on health care, by far the highest in the world.[56]

The same study, once again by the OECD, found that Germany spent 12.8 percent of their GDP on health care, the second highest percentage. We spend 28 percent more of our GDP on health care than the country that spends the second highest amount in the world, as this chart shows:

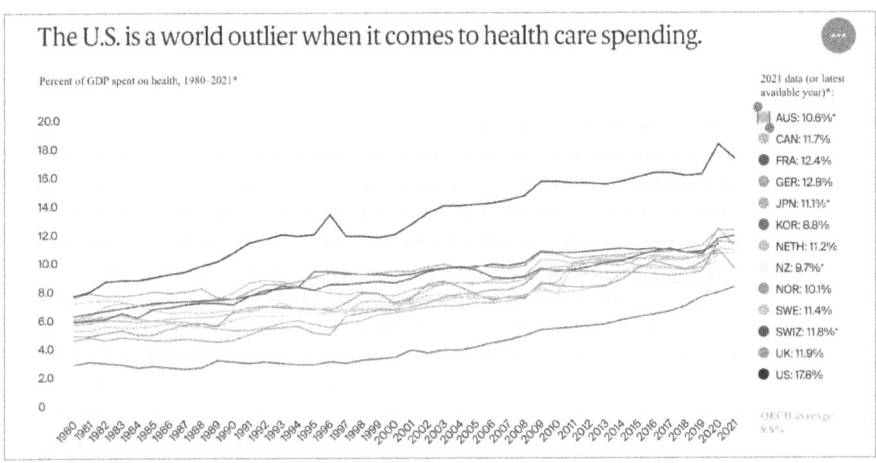

*Fig. 4: Percentage of GDP spent on health care in OECD countries*

---

53 https://www.cms.gov/data-research/statistics-trends-and-reports/national-health-expenditure-data/historical?platform=hootsuite

54 https://www.statista.com/chart/8658/health-spending-per-capita/

55 https://www.oecd-ilibrary.org/sites/675059cd-en/index.html?itemId=/content/component/675059cd-en

56 https://www.statista.com/statistics/184968/us-health-expenditure-as-percent-of-gdp-since-1960/

The next question is this: Given that we pay more than anyone else for it, do we get the best health care in the world in return? Is it commensurate with the amount of money we are spending? Let's take a look.

One way to measure the quality of a country's health care is to look at the average life expectancy of its people. The basic expectation here is that better medical care should yield longer lives.

What, then, is the life expectancy of someone living in the United States compared to those who live in other countries that spend less for their medical care? The picture's not good. Here are the results from a representative handful of the best studies of life expectancy. What needs to be noted here is the timeline. Many of the statistics were gathered from 2016 through 2023. It should be noted that there is a significant decrease in life expectancy in the United States during this period that is not reproduced in the other countries of the world:

1. A United Nations Development Program study found that in 2023 the United States ranked **47th** in the world for life expectancy.[57] The leading country was Hong Kong with a life expectancy of 85.83 years. The second leading country was Macao with 85.51 years, whereas the average expectancy in the United States was only 76.4 years.[58] Germany, the country that spends the second highest amount of money on health care, ranked third with an average life expectancy of 82.18 years.[59] With the adjustments made for the CDC data on life expectancy in the United States as of 2021, the United States falls to a dismal **80th** in the world for life expectancy. Let that sink in for a minute. The following figures illustrate how we are continuing to plummet over time.

---

[57] https://worldpopulationreview.com/country-rankings/life-expectancy-by-country
[58] https://www.cdc.gov/nchs/products/databriefs/db456.htm
[59] https://www.worldometers.info/demographics/life-expectancy/

2. The figures from the World Health Organization for 2016 were comparable. Japan had the highest life expectancy with 83.7 years. Switzerland was second at 83.1 years. The United States was **38th** at 77.8 years.[60]
3. Finally, the figures put together for 2016 by the Central Intelligence Agency of the United States found that the tiny European country of Monaco had the highest life expectancy with 89.4 years! Switzerland was 10th at 82.6 years, and the United States was **57th** at 78.8 years!

More than that, life expectancy in the United States has dropped for the last nine years in a row, from 78.9 years in 2014 to 76.4 in 2023.[61] Statistical analysis has shown that this drop was due to increased numbers of suicides, drug overdoses, alcoholism, and obesity. The last time our life expectancy dropped was during the flu epidemic right after World War I. We are the only developed nation in the world where this is happening. Even the COVID-19 pandemic did not have this kind of impact.

By this one measure alone, it looks as though the United States health care system is not what it should be, especially given what we pay for it. Something seems to be amiss.

But let's not jump to conclusions. Let's take a look at studies that have assessed the quality of health care in nations around the world by taking into account several different aspects of health and health care in each country.

The global Healthcare Access and Quality Index for 2016, published in the leading British journal *The Lancet*, measured the quality of health care in 195 countries.[62] Iceland ranked first, Norway second, and the Netherlands third. The United States ranked **29th**. In a separate study of its own, the World Health Organization ranked our health care system

---

60 https://www.who.int/docs/default-source/gho-documents/world-health-statistic-reports/world-heatlth-statistics-2016.pdf

61 https://www.hsph.harvard.edu/news/hsph-in-the-news/whats-behind-shocking-u-s-life-expectancy-decline-and-what-to-do-about-it/

62 https://www.thelancet.com/journals/lancet/article/PIIS0140-6736(18)30994-2/fulltext

as being the **37th** best in the world.⁶³

The Bloomberg Global Health Index measures the quality of health in countries around the world to see which health care systems give their people the best health. Some of the variables they consider when determining which countries are healthiest include the following:

1. Life expectancy
2. Rates of malnutrition
3. The causes of death
4. The availability of clean water
5. The rates of different risk factors in each country's population (e.g., the use of tobacco, the prevalence of high blood pressure, and the prevalence of obesity)

In the Bloomberg study, Spain ranked first, Italy second, Iceland third, and Japan fourth. The United States was **35th**.⁶⁴

In a 2017 study, the Commonwealth Fund evaluated the quality of health care in 11 developed countries: Australia, Canada, France, Germany, Netherlands, New Zealand, Norway, Sweden, Switzerland, the United Kingdom, and the United States. They measured variables like longevity, the general health of the country's population, how many deaths were caused by inadequate medical care, the affordability of health care, the timeliness with which health care is delivered, and the equity of care by income. Do poor people get the same quality of health care as middle- and upper-class people?

The United States ranked dead last among these 11 countries. The United Kingdom was first, Australia second, and the Netherlands third.

Finally, the OECD has done a series of fascinating studies on the quality of health care by type of disease. For example, they assessed the quality of treatment that patients get for different kinds of cancer in

---

63 https://en.wikipedia.org/wiki/World_Health_Organization_ranking_of_health_systems_in_2000
64 https://www.datapandas.org/ranking/healthiest-countries

different countries, the quality of treatment that patients get for heart attacks, and so forth.

To assess the quality of health care for cancers, the OECD compared the five-year survival rates for several different cancers in several different countries.

Here are the five-year survival rates for breast cancer by country:

**Breast cancer 5-year survival rate**

| Rank | Country | Survival rate | Period |
|---|---|---|---|
| 1 | United States | 88.7% | 2004–2009 |
| 2 | Australia | 87.7% | 2005–2010 |
| 2 | Canada | 87.7% | 2003–2008 |
| 4 | Sweden | 87.4% | 2007–2012 |
| 5 | Japan | 87.3% | 2000–2005 |
| 6 | Iceland | 87.1% | 2007–2012 |
| 7 | New Zealand | 86.4% | 2006–2011 |
| 8 | Israel | 86.2% | 2004–2009 |
| 9 | Norway | 86.1% | 2006–2011 |
| 10 | Finland | 85.9% | 2005–2010 |
| 10 | Netherlands | 85.9% | 2006–2011 |
| 12 | South Korea | 85.2% | 2006–2011 |
| 12 | Slovenia | 85.2% | 2007–2012 |
| 14 | Belgium | 85.0% | 2005–2010 |
| 14 | Germany | 85.0% | 2004–2009 |
| 16 | Singapore | 84.6% | 2006–2011 |
| 17 | Austria | 84.1% | 2007–2012 |
| 18 | Portugal | 82.6% | 2005–2010 |
| 19 | Denmark | 82.0% | 2006–2011 |
| 19 | United Kingdom | 82.0% | 2007–2012 |
| 21 | Czech Republic | 80.7% | 2005–2010 |
| 21 | Latvia | 80.7% | 2006–2011 |
| 23 | Ireland | 80.5% | 2005–2010 |
| 24 | Poland | 73.6% | 2003–2008 |

*Fig. 5: Five-year survival rates for breast cancer by country*

The chart shows that when it comes to the treatment of breast cancers, we are the best in the world, which is encouraging.

However, when it comes to the treatment of cervical cancers, we are not. Here are the five-year survival rates by country for cervical cancer:

| \multicolumn{4}{l}{Cervical cancer 5-year survival rate} | | | |
|---|---|---|---|
| Rank | Country | Survival rate | Period |
| 1 | South Korea | 76.8% | 2006–2011 |
| 2 | Israel | 71.4% | 2004–2009 |
| 2 | Norway | 71.4% | 2006–2011 |
| 4 | Iceland | 70.5% | 2007–2012 |
| 5 | Japan | 70.2% | 2000–2005 |
| 6 | Austria | 67.9% | 2007–2012 |
| 7 | Australia | 67.5% | 2005–2010 |
| 8 | Sweden | 67.3% | 2007–2012 |
| 9 | Netherlands | 66.5% | 2006–2011 |
| 10 | Denmark | 66.4% | 2006–2011 |
| 11 | Belgium | 66.0% | 2005–2010 |
| 11 | Canada | 66.0% | 2003–2008 |
| 13 | Finland | 65.1% | 2005–2010 |
| 14 | Czech Republic | 64.9% | 2005–2010 |
| 15 | New Zealand | 64.7% | 2006–2011 |
| 16 | Germany | 64.5% | 2004–2009 |
| 17 | Portugal | 64.1% | 2005–2010 |
| 18 | Slovenia | 63.0% | 2007–2012 |
| 19 | United States | 62.2% | 2004–2009 |
| 20 | United Kingdom | 60.9% | 2007–2012 |
| 21 | Singapore | 60.6% | 2006–2011 |
| 22 | Latvia | 58.0% | 2006–2011 |
| 23 | Ireland | 57.2% | 2005–2010 |
| 24 | Poland | 52.7% | 2003–2008 |

*Fig. 6: Five-year survival rates for cervical cancer by country*

As you can see from the chart, when it comes to the treatment of cervical cancer, we rank only 19th in the world.

When the OECD evaluated the quality of treatment that we give for heart attacks and strokes, we did better, but we still fell down the list to seventh best. For the treatment of strokes caused by the blockage of an artery that goes to the brain, we ranked fourth. For the treatment of strokes caused by a ruptured artery, we ranked sixteenth in the world.

We Americans pay more than anyone else in the world for our health care, but the quality of the health care we receive in return does not come close to being the best health care in the world.

To complete the picture, let's look at exactly what we are paying for. In 2021 the United States spent more than $4.3 trillion for medical care as calculated by the Centers for Medicare and Medicaid Services.[65] More than $1 trillion was spent on medical care received in hospitals. Another $725.6 billion was spent on medical care received in an outpatient setting, and $335 billion was spent on prescription drugs. Almost $1 trillion was deemed as wasteful, inefficient spending.[66]

When you look at the magnitude of these figures, it is tempting to conclude—as many have—that the most effective way to reduce the cost of our medical care is to simply: (1) reduce hospital costs; (2) reduce doctor fees; and (3) regulate the pharmaceutical industry and make them charge less for their products.

This won't work. Slashing costs will lead to, at best, a modest decrease in the cost of our medical care, but it will not improve the quality of our health care. It is easy to imagine that it might even make it worse.

Even though it might seem to defy common sense, the key to reducing the cost of our health care is to improve the quality of the medical care we're getting. These are lessons I can teach.

The key is chronic illnesses. We can dramatically reduce the cost of

---

[65] https://www.cms.gov/data-research/statistics-trends-and-reports/national-health-expenditure-data/historical?platform=hootsuite

[66] https://www.pgpf.org/blog/2023/04/almost-25-percent-of-healthcare-spending-is-considered-wasteful-heres-why

health care by finding better ways to treat them. Here's why: The bulk of the money we spend on health care in the United States goes toward treating chronic diseases.

The Partnership to Fight Chronic Disease calculates that 90 cents of every dollar we spend on health care each year in the US is for the treatment of chronic diseases alone.[67] The Center for Disease Control (CDC) says that "90% of our health care expenditures are for people with chronic and mental health conditions."[68]

In other words, the reason that health care is so expensive in America is that we spend enormous amounts of money on chronic diseases. Why do we do this?

Because mainstream medicine doesn't know how to cure them, which is, as we've discussed, why they're chronic. These diseases last the length of a patient's life, which is why we spend so much money on them.

In contrast, I can cure chronic diseases, and my methods of treatment are several orders of magnitude less expensive than those of mainstream medicine.

I'm going to spend the remainder of this chapter describing how I treat one specific disease: diabetes.

## THE TREATMENT OF DIABETES

It costs roughly $16,752 per year for mainstream medicine to treat a patient with type 2 diabetes in the United States, and, of course, that's every year for the rest of a patient's life because mainstream medicine doesn't cure diabetes.[69]

If a patient is diagnosed with type 2 diabetes at the age of 40, they may need treatment for another 30 years, maybe even another 40 or 50 years. If the cost of their diabetes treatment somehow remained the same,

---

67 https://www.fightchronicdisease.org/about

68 https://www.healthcentral.com/chronic-health/
the-cost-of-being-chronic-in-2023-a-special-report

69 https://diabetesjournals.org/care/article/41/5/929/36592/
The-Cost-of-Diabetes-Care-An-Elephant-in-the-Room

their diabetes would cost them more than $500,000 over the course of the remaining 30 years of their life—if there are no complications, such as serious circulatory, kidney, heart, and eye problems, which diabetes routinely causes. Almost certainly, complications will add to the lifetime cost of managing a diabetic patient's illness.

Add to this the fact that the Centers for Disease Control issued a report in 2022 that said that 133 million American adults have diabetes or pre-diabetes (almost one-third of the American people), and you can begin to understand why our health care costs amount to more than $4 trillion per year.[70]

My approach to treating diabetes is much different from that of mainstream medicine. I calculate that I can reverse the average case of diabetes in six months to a year for less than what the average patient will spend for one year to manage the condition.

Think about that. In six months to a year, and for less than $16,752, that will be the end of it. There will be no need for any further treatment. No more insulin shots. No more pills. No more endless blood tests to measure the status of your blood sugar. No more worries.

There are two types of diabetes: type 1 and type 2. The cause of type 1 diabetes is your body failing to produce enough insulin, a hormone we all need to be healthy because it causes glucose to move from our bloodstream into our cells. Our cells need glucose for a number of reasons—primarily for energy and the synthesis of other molecules.

If your body doesn't produce enough insulin, the glucose in your body will remain in your bloodstream, and the amount of glucose in your blood will become astronomically high. This increase in blood sugar causes all the problems that occur in diabetes.

The treatment for type 1 diabetes is to take insulin by injection. About 5 percent of all cases of diabetes in America is type 1.

Type 2 diabetes is different. It is caused by a phenomenon called **insulin resistance**, a condition in which your body produces enough

---

70 https://www.cdc.gov/diabetes/data/statistics-report/index.html

insulin but doesn't respond properly to the insulin. The insulin is there, but it doesn't cause your cells to open their doors and allow more glucose to come in as it normally would. As a result, the sugar remains in your blood, and your blood sugar level increases. Now you have diabetes. Ninety-five percent of all diabetes cases in the United States is type 2. It is one of our major health problems.

The mainstay of mainstream medical treatment for type 2 diabetes is to prescribe one of several different types of medications that reduce the level of glucose in your blood in different ways. One medication they use is insulin, which I believe is ridiculous, counterproductive, and even dangerous. Their use of insulin exemplifies much of what they misunderstand about diabetes.

To understand why I insist that insulin should not be given to patients with type 2 diabetes, let's look at my overall view of the physiology of diabetes, which is diametrically opposed to mainstream medicine's view of how the body creates type 2 diabetes.

The best way to explain my view is to start by taking a look at the history of diabetes in America. Since 1970, the number of people with diabetes in the United States has increased dramatically, data backed up by the CDC which has measured the number of people in the USA with diagnosed diabetes for almost all the years between 1958 and 2022.

Below are two charts that illustrate the number and percentage of Americans who had diabetes in the USA for two different periods: 1973-1976 and 2011-2015. These figures show how the rate of diabetes in the USA increased dramatically between these two periods of time.

These CDC figures show that the number of Americans with diagnosed diabetes in 1973 was

**1973-1976**

| Year | Percentage | Number (in millions) |
|---|---|---|
| 1973 | 2.04 | 4.19 |
| 1974 | – | – |
| 1975 | 2.29 | 4.78 |
| 1976 | 2.36 | 4.97 |

*Fig. 7: Number and percentage of Americans with diabetes from 1973 to 1976*

4.19 million; in 2015 the number was 23.35 million. That's sizable growth over the last five decades.

The following graph, also from the CDC, summarizes how the number of cases of diabetes grew steadily in the United States between 1958 and 2015:

**2011-2015**

| Year | Percentage | Number (in millions) |
|---|---|---|
| 2011 | 6.78 | 20.74 |
| 2012 | 6.96 | 21.47 |
| 2013 | 7.18 | 22.30 |
| 2014 | 7.02 | 21.95 |
| 2015 | 7.40 | 23.35 |

*Fig. 8: Number and percentage of Americans with diabetes from 2011 to 2015*

Today the statistics are even more staggering. Diabetes now afflicts 11.3 percent of the population and more than 37.3 million people.[71] These figures underscore a central idea to my vision of both the physiology and the treatment of type 2 diabetes. I believe that there is one very specific reason that the number of people with diabetes has increased so dramatically over the last five decades: The American medical establishment has vilified cholesterol and the triglycerides, insisting that we banish these fats from our diets because they cause hardening of the arteries (atherosclerosis), heart attacks, and strokes. The exile of fat from the American diet started in the 1970s and continues to this day.

It's true that high levels of dietary fat can be associated with heart attacks and strokes, but do those high levels cause these conditions? As we already know, lowering the level of fat in the blood does not significantly decrease the rate of heart attacks and strokes. It does, however, cause insulin resistance and type 2 diabetes.

I have no doubt that the low-fat diet that mainstream medicine advocates is the cause of the epidemic of type 2 diabetes we now face as a nation. Low-fat diets cause insulin resistance every time. Period. This means that they also cause type 2 diabetes because insulin resistance is the physiological cornerstone of type 2 diabetes.

The reason that low-fat diets cause diabetes is that you have to have fats in your diet to regulate blood sugar. If you don't have enough fat in your diet, your blood sugar will go sky high and you will develop insulin resistance. Here's why: We human beings eat foods that belong to the three major food groups: carbohydrates, fats, and proteins. Two of them cause increased insulin secretion and one of them typically does not.

All the carbohydrates that we eat—100 percent of them—are converted into sugar. That means that whenever you eat carbohydrates—pasta, bread, potatoes, fruits, sweets—they will be turned into sugar and increase the amount of sugar in your blood.

Believe it or not, this is also true for protein. Of all the protein that we eat, 58 percent is converted into sugar. So even when you eat meat,

---

71 https://www.cdc.gov/diabetes/data/statistics-report/index.html

you are increasing the amount of sugar in your blood.

This means that whenever you eat carbohydrates or protein, the amount of sugar in your blood will increase. The increased sugar will, in turn, cause your pancreas to secrete more insulin. This is your body's natural response to increased glucose. It gives your cells the glucose it needs, and, at the same time, it reduces your blood sugar. All of this is healthy and good—unless you have elevated levels of sugar in your body for long periods of time.

And this is why a low-fat diet is a problem. A low-fat diet generates high levels of sugar in your blood that persist and remain high for long periods of time. Having persistently high levels of glucose means your cells get overstuffed with glucose and can't take in any more. Regardless, your pancreas will keep secreting insulin because it is trying to lower your blood sugar, but the insulin won't move the excess glucose into your cells because they are already filled to the brim with it.

Mainstream medicine's strategy is to try to push more glucose into a diabetic patient's cells by giving them either insulin or some other medication. But since the cells are already full, the medications don't work. They stop responding to the insulin that would normally move them to take in more glucose. **This is, by definition, insulin resistance**. There is plenty of insulin in your blood, but your cells are not responding to it because they can't.

The end results of this dynamic are: (1) your cells stop taking in glucose; (2) the level of glucose in your blood gets high and stays high; and (3) the level of insulin in your blood continues to rise because your pancreas keeps secreting it, attempting to lower the excessive amount of sugar in your blood.

Now you have type 2 diabetes, a bodily state in which you have too much glucose and insulin in your blood because your cells are unable to open up and take in more glucose.

Mainstream medicine practitioners do not understand this physiology that causes type 2 diabetes. This is why they do not cure it, and this is why they don't understand that the body needs fat to maintain healthy blood sugar levels—which brings us back to why we need fat to prevent type 2 diabetes. When you eat fat, it does not—unlike carbohydrates and protein—increase your blood sugar. It is the only nutrient that doesn't. When you have enough fat in your diet, your body is able get the energy it needs without causing the increase in glucose and insulin levels that carbohydrates and proteins cause.

The key to fixing diabetes is to get more fat into your diet and less sugar. Getting fat into a diabetic patient's diet will give their body the energy it needs without increasing their blood sugar or causing insulin secretion.

However, getting fat into the diet is just one dimension of the treatment I provide a diabetic patient. I give them several modalities of treatment, all of which are necessary. Let's take a look at the larger picture of how I treat a diabetic patient.

## STRESS IS THE CAUSE OF ALL DISEASE

I believe that stress is the cause of all disease. Not some of it. All of it. In my medical universe, there are three categories of stress that cause disease:

1. Mechanical Stresses – including things as varied as accidents, traumas, and injuries

2. Emotional Stresses – including such issues as a sick child, the death of a spouse, an abusive marriage, financial problems, a brutal boss, or any number of other stressful situations, ideas, concepts, or images we believe in as well

3. Nutritional Stresses – including poisons, toxins, and pathogens, things that invade or enter the body (e.g., eating too much sugar, not eating enough fat, not properly digesting any of the three food types and so forth)

***Emotional stress can generate changes in your body that will cause physical illness. Worrying too much might cause an ulcer. Constant arguments with a spouse might cause headaches. Harsh and controlling parents might cause asthma.

I heal my patients by removing all three types of stress from their bodies. The basic idea is that clearing your body of its stresses will restore to it the resources it needs to do whatever needs to be done to naturally heal itself.

To understand how I clear a patient's body of its accumulated stresses, let's take a look at how I treat a diabetic patient. This will show us two things: (1) how I heal my patients; and (2) how my approach to healing dramatically reduces the cost of health care.

## THE TREATMENT OF THE NUTRITIONAL STRESSES IN DIABETES

I give my diabetic patients three basic nutritional treatments to reduce the nutritional stresses that cause diabetes. They are:

1. Timing and an end to snacking
2. Increasing the patient's fat intake
3. Decreasing the patient's sugar and carbohydrate intake

The overall goal of these treatments is to reduce the amount of glucose and insulin in the patient's blood. Once you accomplish this, the insulin resistance that causes type 2 diabetes will disappear, and the patient will be cured.

This is entirely different from mainstream medicine's approach. For one, my approach does not involve taking any medications, whereas the mainstream approach is centered around medications.

Secondly, mainstream medicine's approach to treating type 2 diabetes is insulin-centric. It tries to either: (1) increase the amount of insulin in the patient's bloodstream; or (2) increase the effectiveness of the insulin already present in the bloodstream. This approach doesn't work because the patient's cells are already full of glucose and have become resistant to the action of insulin.

Here is the kicker: When you keep giving insulin to a type 2 diabetic, the insulin becomes "toxic." The excess glucose in the blood gets routed to the liver where it is converted into fat. The excess fat causes a disease of the liver known as fatty liver — a condition in which too much fat is stored in the liver, causing a disease called cirrhosis of the liver. When a patient has cirrhosis, the cells of the liver die and are replaced by scar tissue. A liver with cirrhosis is a liver loaded with scar tissue. If you have cirrhosis of the liver, you are really sick. This is the same liver disease that kills alcoholics.

This brings us back to the three nutritional treatments that I administer to my diabetic patients.

Depending upon carbohydrates for your energy ultimately results in higher levels of sugar and insulin in your blood—a vicious cycle that causes insulin resistance and type 2 diabetes. The cure for this vicious cycle is to simultaneously increase your fat intake and reduce your sugar and carbohydrate intake. The fat you eat will give your body energy, which will allow you to reduce the amount of sugar and carbohydrates you eat. This will, of course, also reduce the amount of insulin your pancreas secretes. Your body will get the energy it needs without increasing the amount of insulin or glucose in your blood.

To help matters along, I recommend two additional measures. One, of course, is to significantly reduce the amount of sugar and starch in your diet. The second measure is the timing of meals and putting an end to snacking. This is very important. If you stop eating between meals, these will become periods of **time** in which you won't be adding any glucose or secreting any insulin into your bloodstream, helping your body lower the amount of insulin in your blood and bringing an end to insulin resistance—the prerequisite for type 2 diabetes.

Finally, even though changing your diet and addressing nutritional issues are central to my approach to treating diabetes, they aren't the whole ball game.

No matter what illness a patient has, I always clear their body of all three types of stress. I do this for two basic reasons: (1) It helps the body heal itself; and (2) the emotional stresses are the cause of many of our chronic physical illnesses.

## THE TREATMENT OF THE MECHANICAL STRESSES IN DIABETES

The body's primary response to all stress is muscle contractions throughout your entire body. This is why you feel tension and pain in your neck, back, and head when you are under stress. That tension and pain are caused by the contraction of those muscles in response to the stress.

Maintaining those contractions is a drain on the body's energy and resources, and this compromises the body's ability to heal itself. If your body is putting its resources into maintaining and coping with stress-induced muscle contractions, it will have less of the resources it needs to keep itself healthy. This is why I clear muscular stress and contractions from the bodies of all my patients—including diabetics.

The second reason I always clear muscle contractions is that the contractions themselves can cause illness. The brain is constantly sending out impulses to all the organs in your body to regulate their activity and maintain your health. Muscle contractions block the transmission of those impulses and make your body sick.

By relaxing those contractions, I restore the brain's ability to communicate with your body and maintain its health. I use the adjustment techniques of chiropractic to relax the muscles contracted by stress. Doing this accomplishes three things: (1) I prevent those contractions from causing illness elsewhere in the body; (2) I free up the body's resources so that the body can balance itself and bring itself back to health; and (3) you feel better because the pain caused by the tension in your muscles is relieved.

There is one more thing about the muscle contractions: They have diagnostic implications. If you know how to read them, they tell you where a person is either sick or in danger of getting sick because a given illness typically causes specific muscles to contract. For example, if a patient has diabetes, the muscles between their shoulder blades will always be contracted. This includes the rhomboid muscles, the trapezius muscles, and the vertebral muscles—the muscles that support your backbone and make it move.

So if I find that a patient has a contracted rhomboid muscle (the muscle that connects your shoulder blades to your backbone), I immediately consider the possibility that the patient has diabetes. However, the rhomboids are not the only muscles I use to make diagnoses. Several other muscle contractions have diagnostic significance as well, and we will take a look at them in the next chapter.

## THE TREATMENT OF THE EMOTIONAL STRESSES IN DIABETES

Emotional stress in and of itself can cause type 2 diabetes. That's right. Emotional stress itself can directly cause insulin resistance, leading you to develop type 2 diabetes even if you are eating well. I know this from my experience working with diabetic patients. This is not a theory.

How in the world, you might ask, does emotional stress cause type 2 diabetes? The answer begins with this fact: When you are in a stressful situation, your body mounts a physiological response to that stress so that you will have the resources to deal successfully with the situation.

If you are descending from a mountain peak in Colorado, and a black bear suddenly clambers up over the south side of the ridge and stands in your way, your body will mount a stress response that will prepare you to deal with the situation: Your heart will quicken and feel like it is trying to jump out of your chest. You will start breathing rapidly. You will feel stronger. Your attention will be riveted to the danger in front of you. Your mind will not wander. This is all part of the fight-or-flight response, which is set in motion by the secretion of different hormones into your blood by the pituitary and adrenal glands and by a part of the brain called the hypothalamus.

One hormone that plays a central role in arousing the body to prepare for either fight or flight is **cortisol**, which is secreted by the adrenal gland (as is adrenalin, another stress hormone). The increased secretion of cortisol into your blood is a normal part of your body's response to a stressful situation. Its purpose is to give you the extra energy you will need to deal with the situation at hand. Cortisol gives you that additional energy by causing your body to synthesize more glucose. Putting extra glucose into your bloodstream is like adding gasoline to your car's tank. It gives you the fuel and energy you need to move around and do things.

Now imagine you are in this situation with the bear. He stands there, 10 feet away from you, slobbering drool that stretches all the way from his mouth down to the ground, which you know is a sign he is ready to attack. (He is drooling over the prospect of eating you.) You quietly tell the bear you are sorry you have intruded into his territory. You tell him you don't mean any harm; you were just having a good time scrambling up Mount Elbert.

The bear turns away and seems to be leaving. Then he turns back and starts to come towards you. Then he turns away again. He goes through this cycle several times, drooling and growling all the while.

During this whole episode, I guarantee you that your cortisol level will be sky high. But when the bear finally turns away for the last time and retreats down the south side of the ridge, the adrenalin and cortisol levels in your blood will return to normal. The bear is gone. The **stress** has passed. There is no longer any need to prepare to fight or flee.

Now imagine that you are in a different kind of stressful situation—a bad marriage. You and your spouse are constantly having bitter arguments—even in front of your kids. Sometimes it gets physical. Sometimes you threaten to leave, and this goes on and on, day after day after day. This stressful situation will also cause your body to push additional cortisol into your bloodstream, just as it would if you ran across a bear on Mount Elbert.

However, there is one important difference between these two situations. When the bear turned and went away once and for all, your body returned to normal. It stopped preparing you to fight or flee, and the level of cortisol in your body returned to its normal level. In the midst of a bad marriage, the situation is entirely different. The level of cortisol in your body will remain high for days and months and years on end because you are constantly suffering from the stress being caused by your marriage.

This kind of chronic response to stress is not unique to a bad marriage. Your body will do the same thing in response to any number of stressful situations, be it financial collapse, working three jobs to make ends meet, the loss of a loved one, a divorce, a child who is constantly getting into trouble with the law, etc.

Chronic emotional stress can keep your body on edge for long periods of time, which means your adrenal glands will continuously secrete excess cortisol into your bloodstream day in, day out. Your body is acting as though you are constantly in the midst of a dangerous fight or flight situation, even though there is no bear there!

This excess cortisol will make your body produce excess glucose for long periods of time, which will cause your pancreas to continuously secrete insulin, and the vicious cycle that generates insulin resistance will begin. Your cells will become overstuffed with glucose, and you will develop type 2 diabetes.

In a nutshell, this is why emotional stress causes 80 percent of all type 2 diabetes cases. More than that, emotional stress causes 80 percent of all our disease.

This is why I always investigate and help clear the emotional stresses from the bodies of all my patients, not just those with type 2 diabetes.

Now let's take a quick look at how I clear the body of emotional stress. (We'll take a systematic look at how I do it in the next chapter.)

I start the emotional work with the premise that the human mind—

through the mechanism of autosuggestion—creates ideas that can get implanted in a person's unconscious or subconscious mind and make them physically sick. This is something I learned from the great mid-20th century Texas chiropractor Dr. Thurman Fleet.

An autosuggestion can be a very specific idea: You are going to have a heart attack one of these days while you are jogging. Or it can be a more general idea, such as one that makes you develop an ulcer because it makes you afraid of life.

Scientific studies have proven that unconscious ideas do indeed cause physical illness. Think back to the research on fixed ideas done in Europe in the second half of the 19th century that we discussed in Chapter 2. Remember the great French neurologist Jean-Martin Charcôt, who showed that a post-hypnotic suggestion—an idea implanted in the mind—can cause the paralysis of a man's arm? That research shows that the fixed ideas in the mind can cause physical illness. Thoughts become things!

I have developed a repertoire of techniques that give me the ability to find and remove these pathogenic fixed ideas from a patient's unconscious mind, which has become the cornerstone of the treatment I now provide my patients.

These techniques work. I've cured many patients by clearing their subconscious mind of a fixed idea that was causing a physical illness. Once the pathogenic fixed idea is cleared from the patient's mind, the illness is often reversed.

In the next chapter, we will discuss at length the techniques I use to clear the fixed ideas that cause illness from a patient's body, but before that, I want to return to and reiterate the central idea of this chapter.

## THE BEST WAY TO REDUCE THE COST OF HEALTH CARE

Health care in America costs way too much. The cost of medical care has bankrupted many people and many families in our country. Most of us, experts and patients alike, look at this picture and call for a straightforward reduction in the cost of medical care. Cut the fees that hospitals charge for rooms, MRIs, and surgeries. Cut the fees that private doctors are allowed to charge for their services. Regulate and reduce the price of our medications. And so forth.

But the larger question is this: What is the best way to cut the cost of medical care? Should we simply slash the costs of mainstream medical care we are receiving now? This won't work, and it is easy to imagine that it might reduce even further the quality of the medical care we are receiving.

Reducing costs might force you to spend fewer days in the hospital after a surgery. Or maybe you won't get all the tests you need. Or maybe you won't get that newer, more expensive—and better—medicine. This is not the right way to go.

My approach to medical care offers us a better solution. My approach to treating chronic diseases provides us with a means to dramatically reduce the cost of medical care while at the same time improve its quality.

Look at the comparison we just made of the costs of medical care for diabetes. I can *reverse* diabetes for a fraction of the cost that mainstream medicine charges to *manage* diabetes for years and decades. This case study shows us how to both reduce the cost of medical care in our country and get better medical care.

As already mentioned, the health care that mainstream medicine gives to diabetic patients costs approximately $16,752 per year—if there are no complications, and if there are no crises that require admission to a hospital. And, of course, diabetic patients receiving mainstream treatment will need to continue getting their treatment for the rest of their life. Over 30 years that will cost the patient $500,000. Over the course of 40 years, that will cost $670,000.

Plus, these patients are not being cured. If you take insulin, you are managing your disease. This is not health. Health is when the disease goes away.

Everything is entirely different for diabetics under my care. For one, I fix my patients! It takes me an average of six months to a year to reverse a diabetic case, and it costs less than $16,000 for the entire treatment. That's it. It's all over for a cost of less than $16,000 versus a cost of several hundred thousand dollars over a lifetime.

This is the remedy for reducing the mammoth costs of health care in America: change the kind of medical care we are giving ourselves. Use mainstream medicine for the illnesses that it treats successfully. Use the kind of medical care I offer for the remaining 80 percent of our illness. This will dramatically reduce the cost of our health care in our country, and it will give us better health care as well!

## CHAPTER 5

# THE DIFFERENCE BETWEEN ME AND MAINSTREAM MEDICINE

*"Hippocrates said, 'Do no harm.' Somewhere between bloodletting and billion-dollar pharma, they got that revised to, 'Do no harm…unless it's covered by insurance.'"*

—Dr. Seán E. McCaffrey

I want you to know that I don't work miracles … yet. What I am doing is fixing people, lots of people, that mainstream medicine is not able to help. I help the patient to turn chronic conditions and disorders into the ghosts of Christmas past. That includes (to name a few):

- Asthma
- Rheumatoid Arthritis
- Endometriosis
- Osgood–Schlatter Disease
- Diabetes
- Ulcerative Colitis
- Psoriasis

In this chapter, we're going to take a look at what makes me unique. There are two fundamental differences between my approach to healing and mainstream medicine's. We are going to look at them one at a time.

## I. CHASING DISEASES VERSUS RESTORING THE BODY'S ABILITY TO HEAL ITSELF

Mainstream medicine chases diseases. What do I mean by that? When you go to see a mainstream medical doctor, they focus on your disease, your illness. They assume you have a disease, and they set out to find what it is and treat it.

Surely that sounds like the right thing to do, doesn't it? This is what we expect of our doctors; and, for some of our illnesses, this approach works. For example, if you have bacterial pneumonia, your mainstream doctor will do quite well for you by focusing on your disease.

The first thing your doctor will do is take your vital signs and ask you to tell the story of what has happened to you. They will ask you when you first started getting sick, and to describe your symptoms.

If you have bacterial pneumonia, you will tell your doctor that you have a high fever, you are coughing a great deal, you are coughing up blood along with green-colored sputum, and you have no energy or appetite. In fact, you have been spending all day in bed.

Any doctor who hears this story will immediately suspect that you have pneumonia, and they will do a series of tests to determine if you do. At the same time, they will also do tests to see if you have some other illness instead.

They will listen to your lungs with a stethoscope to see if they have the characteristic sounds of pneumonia. They will do a chest X-ray to see if it shows pneumonia. They will do a blood test to see if your white blood cells are elevated. They will have their laboratory look at your sputum under a microscope and culture it to see if there are any bacteria present in your lungs, and if so, what kind of bacteria.

This last step—the sputum culture—is very important. It tells your doctor what kind of antibiotic to give you. Different antibiotics kill different bacteria, and you have to get the right one to be cured.

This is all done to determine exactly what disease you have. In other words, your mainstream doctor is entirely focused on finding your disease. This is the first aspect of "chasing diseases."

The second aspect is that mainstream doctors focus on treating your disease. This must seem, once again, like the right thing to do. Of course you want your doctor to treat and cure your disease. This happens to us all the time. We go to see our doctors about a disease, and we get treated for that disease. What could possibly be wrong?

If you have meningitis, you get an antibiotic. If you have chest pain caused by hardening of the arteries, you get your coronary arteries cleaned out. If you have cancer, you have the cancer removed and/or killed with radiation or chemotherapy. Of course this is the right thing to do.

Not so fast.

Remember this crucial fact: 70-80 percent of all our illnesses are chronic illnesses that mainstream medicine is unable to cure. "Chasing" these diseases is not the right thing to do. So what do I do if not chase diseases?

I set the body free so that it can heal itself. It almost doesn't matter what disease a person has. I'm not about curing diseases. I set the body free by doing one specific thing: I remove as many stresses as possible from a patient's body and life.

Think of it like this: Suppose you are climbing Mount Everest—the highest mountain in the world. If you try to climb Everest with 100 pounds of gear and food in your backpack, you are not going to make it to the top. Not even a Sherpa can summit Everest with 100 pounds on their back. However, if you carry only 20 pounds, and if you are in good shape and have the requisite mountaineering skills, it is much more likely that you will succeed and summit Everest (especially if you have a Sherpa helping you get to the top!).

It is the same with your body when you are fighting off an illness. If you are carrying several different types of stress in your body, it will not be able to heal itself because it is spending too much of its energy and resources dealing with those stresses. However, if you are not carrying around a load of stresses in your body, it will have the resources it needs to defend itself against any kind of stress or illness that you might develop.

According to my reckoning, the average human being is always carrying several different stresses within their body. Even the happiest of people experience stress. Gravity is a stress, always pulling away at your body, and, although we are unaware of it, it takes energy and muscle work to keep ourselves from falling to the ground.

Another example of a stress is an injured toe. In my experience, an injured toe is a stress that can cause a heart attack. Wait a minute. Injured toe? Heart attack? Really?

Here's how it works. If you have an injured toe, it can cause your soleus muscle—a muscle in your lower leg—to adapt to the injury by taking on a new shape or function. In a healthy body, the soleus muscle plays a large role in pumping blood back from your feet up to your heart. When it reconfigures itself to deal with the toe pain, its ability to pump blood back to your heart is compromised and reduced. With less blood returning to the heart, the heart can fail, or you can even have a heart attack.

The basic principle at play here is that a stress in one part of your body can cause inflammation and illness—even severe illness—in another part of your body. You stub your toe on the piano. You change your posture to reduce the pain. Your soleus muscle changes its configuration, and, the next thing you know, you have a heart problem.

By removing stresses from a patient's body, I can both prevent disease and cure it—I help the body heal itself.

I removes stresses in a number of different ways. These might include, for example, releasing tension in the muscles that encircle and hold up your backbone, increasing your dietary fat intake, clearing the emotion congestion from your body that is causing a liver disease, or removing an idea from your subconscious mind that is causing a cancer or an endometriosis.

## M.E.N. ARE THE CAUSE OF ALL DISEASE

I do this because my work proceeds on the premise that the human body has a native intelligence that it uses day in, day out to naturally heal itself—if it has the necessary resources to do so.

An obvious example of the body's natural ability to heal itself is the immune system, which we all have within us and which naturally fights off infections. It's a collection of white blood cells, antibodies, and messenger molecules. The inflammatory response is another of many systems that the body uses to help itself fight off disease.

This is why I heal my patients by removing the stresses in their bodies. Once the body is liberated from the stresses that are hiding in it, it will have the resources it needs to heal itself.

What, then, is stress? And how does it rob the body of its ability to heal itself?

The word stress can be a bit confusing because it has two completely different meanings, both of which are true, and both of which are relevant to understanding how I heal my patients.

One meaning of stress refers to stressful situations: a traffic jam when you are rushing to get to the airport to catch a plane, a bad marriage, losing your job, a doctor telling you that you have cancer, climbing Mount Everest, finding yourself in a dark alley at night in Baghdad with three large, armed men coming your way.

The second meaning of stress refers to the way your body responds to stressful situations. If you find yourself in that dark alley in Baghdad, your body will set in motion several different processes that will prepare you to deal with the situation—to either fight those men or turn around and run for your life.

We have talked about these preparatory processes before. They are initiated by hormones secreted by the brain, pituitary gland, and adrenal gland; and these hormones ready you to either fight the environmental stress coming your way or to flee from it. Fight or flight.

The exact same sequence of bodily processes will unfold in response to every stressful situation you encounter—a bear attack, a dark alley, playing football in front of 70,000 people, or climbing a scary mountain.

Scientist Hans Selye studied the sequence of processes that the body mounts in response to stress. He mapped out all the steps that take place as your body responds to a stressful situation, and he gave that sequence a name: the general adaptation syndrome (GAS). Understanding the GAS will help us grasp why the body's stress response both causes disease and keeps your body from healing itself naturally.

As Dr. Selye defined the GAS, it unfolds in a sequence of three phases in response to a stressful situation: the alarm phase, the resistance phase, and the exhaustion phase. I've built upon Selye's theory of stress and believe that there are six, not three stages. They are as follows:

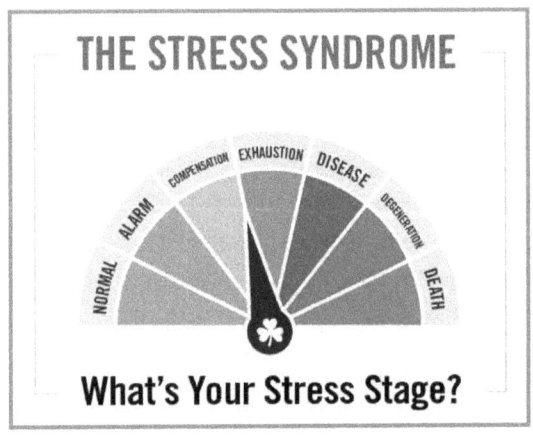

## A. THE NORMAL PHASE

The body starts out in this phase, feeling no pain or discomfort. You sleep well, feel mentally alert, and live an active and vibrant life. Then, for one reason or another, a stress enters your life!

## B. THE ALARM PHASE

It could start with a simple fall, an acute trauma, or simply leaning on your arm until it falls asleep. Your body goes through the alarm phase hundreds—if not thousands—of times every day. Most of the time you are completely unaware of it. The body resists the stress and returns to normal. However, sometimes the stress is too constant or too great for the body to easily adapt so it moves into the next phase: the resistance phase.

## C. THE RESISTANCE PHASE

Your body starts to resist the stress by trying to remove it, usually with muscle contractions that can go on for seconds to a year or more with moderate symptoms. However, if the stress is not removed, the time will come when your body is no longer able to resist it without injuring itself. Consider this analogy I use when explaining this concept to my patients. Try it for yourself and see the effects stress can have on the body.

Squeeze your hand closed into a fist. Squeeze it tighter and tighter. Now hold that for the next four days! My patients usually chuckle when I tell them to imagine this. When I ask them what would happen if they really had to perform such a task, patient after patient notes how tired the hand would become. At this point, the body enters the next phase: the exhaustion phase.

## D. THE EXHAUSTION PHASE

Maybe your body has been suffering for decades or the stress was so great that your body has been suffering for only moments. Either way, it has been trying to resist the stress but has run out of resources and lacks the energy to fight back. Body tissue starts to fail as your body tries too hard to adapt. At this point, the body enters the exhaustion phase, bringing with it a host of noticeable symptoms that could include hormonal imbalances, inflammation, ulcers, depression, insomnia, and more.

The unique attributes of the exhaustion phase are that no pathology—as defined by medicine—is present yet, which means that your physician lacks sufficient evidence to diagnose your condition and sends you home without options. No X-ray, CAT scan, or blood test will detect the tissue failure that is happening. It's too soon for a mainstream medical doctor to diagnose it. This is a critical point in my care. Symptoms abound but no tests are able to validate them. It is at this point that I feel so many of today's illnesses could be reversed or avoided if you only knew how to look for the telltale signs. Lacking this knowledge, the body merely progresses into the next phase: the disease phase.

## E. THE DISEASE PHASE

If left untreated, exhaustion gives way to disease. The exhausted tissues in your body can no longer resist the stressors, and they become diseased. Your body has been forced to permanently change and compensate in ways that are much less perfect. Now your doctor's standard medical tests can effectively demonstrate how badly things are damaged. Symptoms quickly become chronic, never seeming to resolve, despite the ever-growing list of prescription medications in your cupboard. Conditions worsen and your body spirals farther out of control into a permanently changing environment of the next phase: the degeneration phase.

## F. THE DEGENERATION PHASE

If left untreated or simply masked with inadequate treatment, the disease state progresses into a state of degeneration as the cells of the body start to permanently change. Body tissues are no longer normal and begin to take on uncharacteristic shapes and functions as the body desperately tries to survive. Often it is to no avail and the body enters the final phase: death.

In essence, these stages tell us two important things about how our bodies get sick when they are faced with a chronic stressor:

1. The body's response to a situational stress, the GAS, can damage the body it is trying to protect if it is not able to successfully remove the original stress to which it is responding.
   For example, if you are in a stressful marriage, your body will keep mounting a stress response to your relationship with your spouse, but of course the biological stress

response occurring within your body is not going to be able to improve your marriage. What it will do, however, is damage your body.

2. If your body's stress response cannot successfully bring an end to a stressor, it will cause your body's organs to become exhausted and diseased and can even result in death.

The stress response is designed to deal with short-term emergencies. You encounter a bear and your body goes haywire, but when the bear finally trots off down the other side of the ridge, your body returns to normal right away. Your fight-or-flight response ceases and comes to a halt. It takes a massive amount of energy and resources to maintain the GAS for a long period of time, and when the stress response goes on for years and years, it causes biological stresses within the body, and eventually they will cause tissue damage, disease, and even death.

Because I focus on removing the stresses in your body caused by the stress response to external stresses, I bring those stress responses to an end, stopping the tissue damage they are causing. This also sets the body free to heal itself.

This is why my healing techniques work so well. I scan your entire body, taking an inventory of the stresses in your body, and I remove as many of them as possible.

This has two fundamental positive effects: It stops the damage being done by the stress response, and it frees up the energy and resources that the stress response was consuming so that your body can use them to restore your health instead.

This is what I mean when I say I don't chase diseases. I don't focus on treating specific diseases as mainstream medical doctors do. Instead, I remove the stresses in your body so that the body can heal itself, a profoundly different approach to healing than that used by mainstream medicine. And I get extraordinarily good results with it.

## II. HEALING CHRONIC DISEASES BY HEALING THE MIND

Imagine for a moment that you are working for a political campaign that has daily group meetings to brainstorm and hash out strategy. It is a Monday morning, and, after having the afternoon off on Sunday, you arrive at the office just before eight. As soon as you get in the door, you are immediately told to join a meeting already in progress with 10 other people.

As you walk in the door, the first person you run into says, "Are you okay? You look sick." The next person says, "Is something wrong?" Then as you take your seat at the conference table, the person to your right turns to say hello, and they look taken aback before saying, "Oh my god. What happened?" Slowly but surely, everybody else chimes in and asks with genuine concern if everything is all right with you.

It is easy to imagine that a person in this situation might end up feeling that something must really be wrong with them. You decide that something actually is wrong with you, and soon thereafter you come down with the flu.

I use this scenario to illustrate how an idea can get implanted in a person's mind and cause both stress and illness. This is an "autosuggestion," a process in which we make up an idea about ourselves that causes us to get sick because of something that has happened to us; it might be something ordinary or it might be something truly difficult. The resulting pathogenic idea is an autosuggestion, a term I inherited from the great Texas chiropractor Dr. Thurman Fleet.

In the normal course of affairs, we human beings routinely create autosuggestions or someone else creates a suggestion that we buy into. Ultimately, these autosuggestions cause much, if not most, of our chronic illnesses.

An important thing to understand about the pathogenic ideas created by autosuggestion is that they are, more or less, a normal part of life. They happen to all of us, and they can take a number of different forms.

Maybe you are a child and your schoolmates tease or taunt you about being poor and from the wrong side of the tracks, and you form the idea that you are unattractive and stupid because you are poor.

Or maybe your schoolmates make fun of you because your mother is having extra-marital affairs, and you form the idea that both you and your mother are shameful people.

Or maybe your father is constantly berating you because you are not becoming the kind of person that he wants you to be, and you form the idea that you are never going to succeed in life. You are going to be a failure.

Or maybe your wife leaves you, and you decide that you were not man enough to keep her.

Or maybe you fear that a protracted hot spell is going to make you come down with something. Or maybe you believe that you will injure your knees because the sand on the beach on which you are doing daily wind sprints is as firm as concrete. Or maybe you go to work in a dangerous neighborhood, and you carry the idea that sooner or later someone is going to mug you. Or maybe someone at work sells more cars than you do, and you come to fear that maybe you are not such a good salesman after all.

The list could go on and on, so let's consider a concrete example of how a fixed idea can cause physical illness. (We're going to continue with this next scenario for several pages, so please stay with me.)

Suppose you have been married for 36 years, and your spouse—who was the love and light of your life—dies. The loss is a large one for you because it was your spouse who made your life bright and lively. They knew how to have fun, and they drew interesting people into your lives.

You, on the other hand, are a solid human being with oodles of integrity. You are a judge, and everyone respects you for your intellectual acumen and the decency that you show to all the people who come before your bench. But you have never really known how to enjoy life, or how to seek out inspiring experiences on your own. Thank goodness that your spouse knew how. They enriched your life and made you a fuller human being by bringing fun, pleasure, and sanctity into your life. You were lucky, and you knew it. You loved your spouse deeply for all that they added to your life.

Now that they're gone, you are convinced that your life is about to become one long series of gray nights and weekends in front of the television. You are convinced that people loved spending time with the two of you because your spouse was so much fun and so good-hearted; now that they're gone, you settle into the idea that you will be spending most of your spare time home alone. Your children are far away, on the other side of the country and in Europe.

Now that your spouse is gone, who will get you out of bed early in the morning to go see the sun rise and absorb its beauty?

The idea takes root in your mind that your life is going to become a joyless marathon to the end.

Before long, these thoughts become a self-fulfilling prophecy. You are spending your nights and weekends in joyless solitude. You start to get depressed. It becomes harder to focus on your work. Your mind wanders, and you find yourself thinking about your spouse when you are hearing cases. You try to find things to do that will keep you busy and give you joy, but they don't seem to be working.

And then, slowly but surely, your body begins to break down even though you are only 58 years old. First you notice that you no longer have the same energy you once had. The next thing you know, you get an ache in your lower back that won't go away. Then you start waking up in the morning with headaches. The quality of your life is going downhill right in front of your eyes. You go to your doctor, and after he X-rays your back and finds nothing, he gives you some painkillers.

Unfortunately, the painkillers cause serious heartburn. To numb the pain and give yourself some kind of pleasure in life, you begin eating far too much. You eat a pint of ice cream with every dinner; and sometimes you throw in some pie or a cake. You snack all day long and start gaining weight, and constipation sets in.

Then comes the final blow. Dementia and angina pectoris. You start forgetting things. Small things at first—dates, appointments, and things you know you have just said. Your colleagues at work begin to notice. You start having the same kind of chest pain that happens when a person has a heart attack. Sometimes you get a pressing pain beneath your chest bone when you are working too hard or going for a walk. You go to see your doctor, and she gives you more medicine.

One day, you stop in front of the full-length mirror in your bathroom and take an honest look at what you have become. You see a tired and joyless old person who is fat, taking lots of medicine, and on the verge of having a heart attack. You feel like you are losing your mind and are scared of what the future might hold.

It dawns on you that you have to reclaim your life and do something about all of this. No one else is going to do it for you.

You go see a friend who is seeing some kind of alternative healer, and you ask how things are going. Your friend tells you that the healer has turned their life around, and that they're healthy again. You get the healer's name and phone number, and you call my office to make an appointment to see me. It is now three and a half years since your spouse passed away.

## YOUR VISIT WITH ME

When we first meet, this is how I want you to see me: I want to blow into the examining room in which you are waiting like a fresh wind. I want you to see that I'm clear-eyed, caring, confident, mildly ebullient, down-to-earth and optimistic.

After asking you a number of questions, I press upon several different points on the back of your skull, which may seem a bit odd to you. After all, no doctor has ever done this before; but several times, when I press on one specific point, it hurts like hell. I know the pain is almost unbearable, even though I don't seem to be pressing all that hard.

Then I ask you to lie on your stomach, and I press on and manipulate the muscles and bones in your back. It will even seem as if I'm moving your vertebrae around a little bit. You can hear them click as I move them into different positions.

Then I ask you to sit up again and I push on that same spot on the back of your head, except now there is no pain. You likely ask me if I'm pressing on the exact same place as before. You're probably wondering why there's no pain. I reassure you that I'm pressing on the exact same point, and you begin to wonder what I did and why the pain is gone.

Next, I ask you to stand up and walk around. You notice that the back pain that you have had for almost three years is much better. It still hurts, but it is nowhere near as bad as it was when you walked in the door. I hope at this point you're thinking, *Hmm, maybe this guy, this alternative healer, really does know what he is doing.*

I finish up this first visit with you by explaining the treatment I've just given you. Before I summarize my explanation, I want to restate the three things I did to you:

1. I pressed on specific points on the back of your skull, and that elicited a great deal of pain.
2. I manipulated and made adjustments to the muscles and bones of your back.
3. I pressed again on the same points on the back of your skull; this time there was no pain.

I begin my explanation of these procedures by telling you that the body's first response to stress is muscle contractions. When the muscles that are wrapped around your backbone contract in response to stress, they cause two additional problems:

1. They can have local effects on the back itself, causing back pain, and they can make your back vulnerable to spasms and injury.

2. They can have distant effects by causing dysfunction in just about any other muscle or organ in your body.

The local effects are simple to understand, but how in the world do muscle contractions in your back cause organ dysfunction elsewhere in your body? This is just as hard to believe as a bum toe causing a heart attack.

The answer is this: When the muscles attached to your spine contract in response to stress, they interfere with the signals the nerves are attempting to send to the brain in response to the stress. The brain is constantly sending signals in the form of nerve impulses out to your entire body. Some of the signals go to your muscles, and some of them go to the organs of your body.

The signals sent out by the brain travel down into your spinal cord along nerves, and they leave the spinal cord along different nerves that go to different destinations in your body. The nerves carry the brain's signals to your muscles and organs, just as electrical lines carry electricity from a power plant to your home.

The nerves leave the spinal cord in clusters. The point at which a cluster of nerves leaves the spinal cord is called a spinal root. There are 31 pairs of spinal roots located all along the length of the spinal cord, and a single nerve root contains nerves that go to several different muscles and organs. When the muscles attached to your backbone contract, they can press upon a spinal root; as they do so, they compromise the function of the nerves that pass through that root.

For example, if a muscle inhibits the nerve that makes the deltoid muscle contract, it will cause the deltoid to have frequent spasms or become weak.

Or if a muscle contraction interferes with the nerve that controls the functioning of the pancreas, it will cause dysfunction in the pancreas. Or if a muscle compresses the nerve that innervates the stomach, it can cause the stomach to have problems. And so forth. **In other words, when the muscles in your backbone tighten in response to a**

**stress, they can cause distant muscles, tissues, organs, and systems to fail and become sick.**

Next I explain to you that the body has six different organ systems that it can and does deploy to respond to a stressful situation. Sometimes it uses one system, sometimes another one, and sometimes it deploys several systems at a time.

Each of these systems is a collection of organs and functions within the body: the glandular system, composed of the endocrine glands; the eliminative system, composed of the sinuses, lungs, skin, bladder, kidneys, gastrointestinal tract, and lymph nodes; the nervous system, which also responds to stress, and so forth.

Each of these organ systems is set in motion and governed by instructions that it receives from specific areas within the brain. Each of these six brain regions is, in turn, connected by nerves to ligaments and tendons attached to one specific point on the nuchal lines that run across the back of the skull. The nuchal lines are a set of small, bony ridges that protrude out just a tiny bit from the occipital bone, the bone that forms the rear portion of the skull.

Each of the six stress response systems is connected to a specific area on the nuchal lines. There is a zone for the glandular system, a zone for the digestive system, a zone for the elimination system, and so forth. In other words, each of the stress response systems is connected to an area in the brain, and then through that brain area to one specific point on your nuchal lines.

When a stress response system is called upon to respond to a stressful situation that a person is stuck in for a long time—say, an unhappy marriage—the organs in that system will become sick because they are being overused and overtaxed. They are going through the exhaustion and disease phases of the GAS.

Here now is the key idea to which we have been building: When one of the six stress response systems becomes dysfunctional because it has exhausted itself as it responds over and over again to a chronic stress, the nuchal tendons and ligaments to which that system is connected will harden and form knots, becoming painful to the touch. When I push on your nuchal lines and find a painful point, that tells me which of your six stress response systems is failing. Those points on the nuchal lines are a diagnostic system that tell me where the stresses are lodged in your body. That's why your skull was painful to the touch—one of your stress response systems was in trouble.

Consider this example: Suppose that I found that the glandular point on your nuchal lines was painful to palpation. This would have told me that there was something wrong with your endocrine glands; but, more than that, it would have also told me how to restore those glands to health. Why? Because for each of the six diagnostic points on the nuchal lines, the stress response system to which that point is attached can be brought back to health by doing adjustments to a specific set of vertebrae in your backbone, removing the obvious stresses and nourishing the body.

In your case, given that you had a glandular problem, there were four specific vertebrae that needed to be adjusted: (1) the first cervical vertebrae; (2) the first thoracic vertebrae; (3) the first lumbar vertebrae; and (4) the sacrum. After I did the adjustments, I went back and pressed the glandular point on your nuchal lines again, and the pain was gone. I had released the contractions in the muscles that were pressing upon the nerves that went to your endocrine glands, restoring the normal flow of brain messages to the glands, beginning the process of restoring them to health. It also released the tension and knots in the tendons connected to the endocrine zone on your nuchal lines. As a result, the nuchal pain disappeared.

The difference is so dramatic that at first you don't believe me. You think that perhaps I was pressing on a different point, but by the time you leave my office, you realize that I had indeed been pressing on the same point, and that something important had happened. It's my hope that you're beginning to think that maybe this "alternative healer" might really be able to help you after all and that you will begin to have faith in me.

Before you leave for home from that first visit, I have you give me a urine sample for a multi-faceted test called the integrated urinalysis panel (IUP).

## YOUR NEXT TWO APPOINTMENTS WITH ME

Your next visit with me begins with the results of the IUP, an important tool in my toolbox. In general, I use it to evaluate two basic aspects of a patient's health: the patient's nutritional status and the resources the patient has been using—and overusing—to fight off the stresses in their body.

Your urine test shows that you're consuming too much sugar and carbohydrates and that you should adjust your dietary intake accordingly. It also shows that you're not digesting your fats properly. I help you correct that by prescribing some enzymes and herbal supplements. I also ask you to alter your diet and stop snacking during the day so that your insulin levels will go down.

Then I repeat the same series of vertebral adjustments that restore the health of the glandular system because it is often necessary to do these adjustments several times to successfully reset a stress response system and return it to health. It is like watering a garden. You don't plant tomatoes today and expect to pick them tomorrow. You care for them. You water them, and in no time you have fruit worth picking.

I finish up our third session by adding a second set of vertebral adjustments to your treatment—the adjustments that will restore your circulatory system to health. Remember, in this scenario, you're suffering from a heart condition—angina pectoris.

Your fourth visit starts out in much the same way. Once again, I examine the nuchal line and do the vertebral adjustments. This time, as I do the adjustments, I explain what I'm doing and why I'm doing it. I name the muscles I'm relaxing, explaining which nerves I'm decompressing and telling you which organs will be returned to health as a result. Most of all, I then describe the healthy state to which your glandular and your cardiovascular systems will return.

Then I give you a piece of paper that describes that healthy circulatory state, and I advise you to read this page out loud to yourself at home several times a day, every day, right before retiring to bed.

I give this same image of perfect circulatory health to all my patients who need it. This is how I describe it:

1. Adjustment of the nerves to the thyroid gland tend to regulate your blood pressure, whether it's too high or too low, because the thyroid regulates your blood pressure.
2. All nerves to the heart are being restored to normal. There will be a change for the better, and you will notice a feeling of ease and strength all over your body.
3. The blood vessels of the back, arms, chest, and abdomen are being brought to normal, and better circulation will naturally result. Aches and pains in these parts will leave, and a feeling of strength and well-being will appear.
4. Blood vessels and lymph vessels of the lower extremity will be brought to normal and you will become aware of more circulation in this area. You will not tire so easily and, in general, will notice more ease of movement in your limbs.

After I finish the vertebral adjustments, I conclude the fourth visit by doing some acupuncture on you to balance the distribution of energy in your body. As I do this, I also begin to ask you more questions about your life and health.

## THE FIFTH VISIT

When you return for your fifth visit, you tell me you're feeling somewhat better. Your energy is beginning to return. You're having less trouble with your stomach. Your constipation is remitting and you notice you're starting to recall things more easily than you have in months.

Now the real work of healing you begins.

I believe that everything that exists in the universe is energy, and, of course, ever since Einstein discovered the special theory of relativity, we have known that this is true.

Einstein's famous equation ($E=mc^2$) can be spelled out to represent that matter can be transformed into energy, and that energy can be transformed into matter. Energy and matter are transformations of one another. For example, atoms of uranium can be split to yield the massive amounts of energy generated by nuclear bombs and nuclear power plants.

Realizing that everything is energy profoundly impacted the way I shaped the treatments that I give to patients who have an illness caused by an emotional stress. I believe that since we are all manifestations of energy, we can form a composite with one another, and through proper suggestion, wrong or harmful concepts can be altered and replaced.

Think, for example, of all the times you have actually felt someone's anger. This is a rudimentary example of how we can receive energy from someone else's mind by accident. It can be infectious and contagious. Especially when the emotions are negative.

I focus on ideas which have unintentionally entered into the subconscious mind to accomplish two basic things: to find and remove the pathogenic fixed ideas causing chronic illnesses, and to help to create positive ideas of health for the mind to focus on to restore health.

I diagnose my patients by finding the fixed ideas causing their illness, and I treat them by both removing the negative ideas and replacing them with the positive ideas of health. The positive images overpower the negative ones, and once they are integrated into the patient's mind, they generate a state of health within a patient's body. Literally, thoughts become things. Ideas in the mind look for expression in the physical body. You get to choose which ideas you wish to feed.

So when you come in for your fifth visit, I begin to create a stronger rapport and a composite with you, both consciously and subconsciously, while doing yet another round of adjustments. I begin asking you a series of questions about your zones so that I can find the fixed ideas and emotions causing your illness.

In this scenario, I start the process by asking you if there are any stressful situations that have caused your illnesses. You say, "Yes." I then ask about an emotional loss or something that might have disrupted your outlook for the future. Did it involve matters of the heart? You are stunned.

Next I ask when this stressful situation occurred. Did it happen within the last five years? "Yes," you say. Did it happen within the last year? "No."

Was it a situation at work? "No." Did the stressful incident involve someone in your family? "Yes." Was it a blood relative? "No." Was it your spouse? "Yes."

Remember, all the while that I'm asking you these questions, I don't know that it was the death of your spouse that set off the chain reaction of thoughts and emotions that had caused all of your illnesses.

At this point, it all comes pouring out of you.

You tell me how wonderful your spouse was and how they opened your life to so many positive things that would never have been part of your life without them. Then you tell me how your life has gone relentlessly downhill ever since they passed away.

I ask your what kind of person you've become since your spouse passed away, and all the negative ideas you attributed to yourself come flooding to the surface. "I am not lovable. People respect me in the legislature, but no one is really drawn to me. I am no fun."

As these ideas come pouring out, I explain to you that these ideas are in part some of the underlying causes of your illness. I go on to say that having these ideas isn't a shortcoming on your part; they are a normal part of life and can happen to anyone.

In this non-judgmental atmosphere, you let go of your negative ideas by ceasing to believe they are true. I guide you to understand how we as individuals get to choose the thoughts and ideas we allow into our minds. We can choose to feed the negative feelings in life or we can feed their opposites.

To reinforce the healing process brought about by this catharsis, I continue to see you several more times. I monitor your diet as you continue to improve it, and I keep doing the adjustments that were curing your glandular and cardiovascular systems because they strengthen and "lock in" the healing concept that I started by clearing your body and mind of the negative pathogenic ideas causing your illness.

In addition, I continue to reinforce the positive ideas of perfect glandular and circulatory health being implanted into your mind. These ideas are important because they generate a state of health and replace the negative ideas that were in your mind before.

With the passage of time, you become healthy again. Your chest pain disappears. You no longer have heartburn. Your energy returns to normal. Your back pain becomes a thing of the past. Your memory returns, and you no longer fear what the future holds.

Most of all, your depression lifts, and you stop thinking that you're uninteresting and unlovable. You begin to reach out to your family and friends once again and develop a rich and rewarding network of friendships.

## ALL THE TREATMENTS

This case study made it possible to show you in depth some of the techniques that I use to heal my patients. However, you should not get the idea that this case study shows you all the diagnostic and treatment techniques I use. I have a much larger repertoire than those I just mentioned. In future books, we will talk about more of them.

You should also know that my approach to healing has evolved over the years. The crux of my healing technique now—especially with patients that have a chronic disease—is to find and remove the fixed unconscious ideas and concepts causing their illnesses because most chronic illnesses are caused by autosuggestions. This does not mean, however, that I no longer use the healing techniques I learned earlier in my career.

When I first came out of chiropractic school, I used two basic healing technologies: the spinal adjustment techniques that form the core of chiropractic therapy and the bag of nutritional treatments I learned from Dr. Loomis. My next step was to try to improve my ability to heal by learning everything I possibly could about nutrition, and to learn several more styles of making chiropractic adjustments. This moved me to next immerse myself in acupuncture and traditional Chinese medicine, and I mastered several different styles of acupuncture. Then I discovered Dr. Fleet's work on autosuggestions.

I have since gone on to have great success ferreting out and clearing away the unconscious ideas and emotions that cause a person to get physically ill. This approach has now become the core of my healing work, though I still use all the healing techniques I learned along the way as well. Why? For two basic reasons.

First, they can provide a patient with immediate relief. The chiropractic adjustments I do can quickly resolve tension and pain in the neck, back, and head. They offer a way to deliver a concept of healing to the patient and help to establish a rapport with the patient that is absolutely critical for patient success. Oftentimes, the nutritional supplements I give my patients further assist the body in rebuilding and repairing systems that have progressed beyond the resistance phase, quickly increasing their energy and relieving their gastrointestinal symptoms.

Secondly, they strengthen the core healing process that I set in motion by clearing a patient's body of its pathogenic ideas and emotions.

I use the earlier methods to relieve the stresses that a patient is carrying around in their body. That frees up the energy and resources that the body needs to carry out the healing process set in motion by removing the pathogenic ideas and emotions from a patient's body. They "lock in" the cure.

This is why every patient that comes to see me now, at this stage in my healing career, will be on the receiving end of all my healing techniques, and they will be much better for it.

# CHAPTER 6

# FROM CONFUSION TO CLARITY: AN IUP EXPERIENCE

*"In medicine, the diagnosis is often a guess dressed in Latin."*

—Dr. Seán E. McCaffrey

There comes the time in everyone's life when they want to do something to make a difference, to make a real change. I have spent the past several decades in search of such a cause, something that I could leave behind that would help humanity elevate itself in one way or another. I began writing this book in March 2019 with that goal in mind: to show society that there was a different way to healing. Along my journey, my knowledge has been refined and polished time and again. I can only hope that I will maintain the desire to learn and evolve my craft until I simply no longer exist in this world. With all of that said, the final chapter of this book is designed to offer a form of self-help to you, the reader.

While thousands of self-help books are currently in publication, I hope my introduction to healing oneself will open up a concept that many of you may have never explored before. The goal of this chapter is to allow you to implement the techniques and theories I'm about to put forward. In doing so, you should make a definite impact on your overall health and well-being. If I accomplish this for you, the entire book was worth writing. It is my sincerest wish that the information I am about to share will help someone change their life for the better.

To proceed, we need to revisit the concept that stress is the cause of all disease and that MEN cause all stress. As I mentioned earlier, stress is the underlying cause of all health conditions—no exceptions. All too often physicians get bogged down in the idea that stress is purely emotional. This is not the case.

Stress comes in three distinct varieties. The M in MEN represents mechanical stress. When my grandfather was in practice, he often referred to this as accidents and traumas. The falls, slips, and major impacts on the body would express themselves here. What needs to be noted at this point is the fact that mechanical stress starts outside and goes into the body—it invades.

The E in MEN represents emotional stress, which comes in two distinct varieties. Quite often your thoughts actually become things. An example of this would be someone becoming angry and their blood pressure elevates. Quite often we will see this in someone who's a chronic worrier. They tend to develop gastrointestinal problems, bowel issues, and ulcers, all of which are physical manifestations of someone's emotional thoughts.

The second variety of emotional stress involves our conscious acts or choices. An example of this might be a diabetic at a party who is confronted with those oh-so-tasty glazed donuts. The diabetic knows donuts are going to aggravate their blood sugar, but they partake in them anyway. Then they are quick to blame the doughnut for their blood sugar being high later on. In reality, the donut had very little to do with this. They chose to eat the donut, knowing that it would aggravate their condition. Millions of people eat donuts every day and are not diabetic. So not only do thoughts become things, but our conscious acts and choices will also manifest in the body physically. A key piece to understanding this side of the triangle is to recognize that your thoughts start inside.

## M.E.N. ARE THE CAUSE OF ALL DISEASE

This brings us to the N in MEN, to nutrition. My grandfather often referred to this side of the triangle as the side of poisons. I chose "nutrition" because I thought MEN was very funny and MEP not so much. To this side we delegate all the poisons, toxins, and chemicals from our environment. Our diet, the things we drink, the air we breathe (or whatever is in the air we breathe), it all falls under this side. All the viruses and bacteria come from outside the body and enter it. They either assist in its function or they interfere with it. Medications, smokes, perfumes, environmental toxins … they all follow the same path.

What I want to point out at this moment is that the nutritional side of the health triangle both starts outside the body and invades it. The emotional side of the health triangle is already inside and therefore must express itself through the other two. Wrong thoughts or wrong acts will express through the body's physical anatomy and to the body's functions such as digestion, elimination, or reproduction, just to name a few. The stresses interfere with normal body processes, and the longer they are allowed to do so, dysfunction will surely begin. If the dysfunction is allowed to persist for an extended period of time, it can eventually evolve into a disease state.

We will begin, then, by observing the four basic laws under which the human body functions best when followed. A brilliant doctor, Thurman Fleet, presented these laws more than 80 years ago, and they are as valid today as they were then. The keyword here is "law." Not "suggestion." Not "recommendation." A *law* regarding how the human body must survive and function. The first of the four laws of the human body is what Dr. Fleet referred to as the Law of Nutrition or Nutrients. It's quite simple in what it states: You have to put the right fuel in the body, in the right combinations, in order for that body to thrive properly. This does not mean you need to be perfect in your dietary selections. But if you could aim for 75 percent then you would be well ahead of the game.

There are literally thousands of diets on the market today, each one claiming that it has figured out the secret to this or that, and therefore, is the only way. After more than two decades in practice and writing numerous weight loss plans for physicians and patients alike, I can assure you there is no "one" way. The human body is masterful at adapting. All one has to do is look around the planet at different cultures in different parts of the world, consuming completely unique and separate diets, and see that they all thrive. The adage "there are many ways to Rome" appears to hold very true when dealing with dietary concerns and nutrition.

There are, however, a few staples that should be acknowledged and adhered to when possible. Simply put, consuming excess sugars and alcohols is fairly hard on the body's digestive and elimination systems. With that said, if I were battling some type of intestinal problem or a stomach disorder, I might consider limiting my sugar intake and alcohol. All too often, we find ourselves getting caught up in looking for the exotic extreme—the unique parasite, the SIBO, the Crohn's, the colitis, the Heliobacter pylori—that we are sure must be the cause of our problem. It could never be excessive overindulgence over long periods of time that led to dysfunction and eventually disease states.

Cleaning up this portion can go a long way. The IUP that we discussed in the previous chapter enables you to take the guesswork out of the nutrition side of the triangle. You no longer have to guess if you're using your carbohydrates, your proteins, or your fats. Are they being absorbed properly? Are your food choices moving through the body efficiently, getting digested, absorbed across the gut wall, and transported to the cell? Are they being utilized by the cell, and is their waste product efficiently being removed so it does not become a poison or a toxin to the rest of the system? The IUP answers all these questions quite convincingly.

This brings me to the second law of the body, the Law of Movement. The human body is designed to move every day, in every way. All one needs to do is look back to a time in their life when they felt well. Quite often it's early childhood or adulthood when we were active, strong, healthy, and vibrant. However, as we age life seems to get in the way. We start taking sedentary jobs, and we no longer play for the joy of it, moving the body all the time, in every way. Little aches and pains start to set in as a result of our lack of use. Once these are established, the pain itself causes us to move even less and, like rust, it starts to spread. But this can be avoided.

Koichi Tohei, the world renowned aikido instructor and energy healer, made multiple mentions of the importance of moving the body every day. He noted the importance of keeping the body strong and flexible. Simple stretches, simple movement of all your parts, often will suffice.

I instruct my patients who have movement issues to start every morning by simply moving the things furthest away from the core. I tell them upon waking to just wiggle their toes back and forth, up and down, 10 to 15 times, and then move their fingers, opening and closing them, back and forth, 10 to 15 times. Next, I tell them to proceed up toward the core of the body and start rolling their ankles while they're in bed and to roll their wrists to accompany that movement, back and forth, in small circles clockwise and counterclockwise. Next they should move up to the next joints, their knees and elbows, opening and closing them gently in small little circles 10 to 15 times. I tell them to work their way up to their hips, rocking them side to side in the bed; then to move their shoulders in circles, back and forth, while lying in bed. Finally, I tell them to work their way to their neck and head, turning their head gently side to side and then looking up and down, up and down, like they have a marker on the tip of their nose and are drawing circles on the ceiling, clockwise and counterclockwise, before they ever get out of bed in the morning.

Simple little movement exercises such as these can be game changers for a body that has become brittle, stiff, achy, and full of inflammation. Movement means to circulate, and proper circulation is absolutely critical for human existence. While there are numerous other beneficial exercises and movement therapies, something this basic can go a very long way.

I have found the use of a slant board to assist in restoring proper posture, balance, and coordination to be essential in my patients' care over the years. Dr. Zhu was critical in my understanding of the use of this device. Used properly, this therapeutic tool can assist weight loss, improve posture, or even calm an angry mind. It is an invaluable tool and serves the Law of Movement very well.

The third law of the body is the Law of Recuperation. It comes in three flavors, very much like the stress triangle. The law simply states you must sleep properly. Those with sleep apnea, those with insomnia—those who cannot sleep at night, who wake anxiously evening after evening—or those who simply sleep way too much are all violating this law.

Now, authorities differ greatly on what is needed for proper sleep. I think it is safe to say that the amount of time the human body needs for proper repair varies depending on what phase of life we're in and the stresses we are under. In 1900, the average amount of sleep that people received in the United States was nine hours per night. As of today, that has decreased to less than six. Just imagine cleaving off a third of your sleep time.

It's important at this stage to acknowledge what sleep actually does. Physiologically, we know that, during sleep, your senses tend to shut down and rest. Your brain goes through a house-cleaning effect. It starts to heal and repair so it can keep the body functioning throughout its waking hours. If we lose a third of our cleaning hours, it's only a matter of time before dysfunction sets in, and we stated above dysfunction often leads to disease. I have wondered many times over the last few decades in practice if the rapid increase in Alzheimer's disease and dementia was the result in some way or another of our altered sleep patterns.

The second phase of recuperation is rest. Rest and sleep are not the same thing. When you sleep, you are completely unaware of your environment and you are recharging the brain's batteries. When you rest, you are simply taking it easy for a few moments throughout your day to allow the body to recover temporarily so you can push on. This function is absolutely critical for day-to-day use and survival. The body needs a little downtime. A small 20-minute nap or often just sitting down to relax for a few moments serves us very well.

Now we must look at the final phase of the Law of Recuperation: the human body's need for recreation—quite often the most overlooked piece of this law. Look at your happy times. Look at your moments that you enjoyed the most in your life. Quite often they are full of you doing something that you enjoy that makes you feel good. Vacationing, traveling, playing sports, maybe reading a book, or simply enjoying your children or your loved ones all give us joy. These all fall under the definition of recreation. We just need to have fun! Puppy's play, kittens play, children play, and they all seem to be healthy and happy. We just need to go back to our childhood and play. The Law of Recuperation is one of my personal favorites for this very reason.

We now are at the final of the four laws of the human body, the Law of Sanitation. On the surface, the Law of Sanitation seems quite obvious. Proper hygiene has done more to eradicate disease on this planet than any vaccination, shot, pill, or potion ever will. Plagues, outbreaks, and diseases of all kinds are often squashed under proper sanitation. Clean water supplies, the proper handling of food, and washing the body every day from head to toe serve as wonderful ways to keep the body refreshed, invigorated, and healthy. It would seem like common sense in today's society, but it really depends on which part of the world you are from and your upbringing.

Are you fortunate enough to have food, clothing, and shelter? Do you live with at least some excess, where water and common things that we often take for granted are not even a thought for you? Or do you find yourself with an illness or an injury that interferes with your ability to properly clean and sanitize the body? (This alone can prevent tremendous amounts of discomfort, dysfunction, and disease in the human body.)

But the Law of Sanitation goes a step further. It is not only referring to the physical body, it is also referring to the mind. Thoughts become things, as we discussed above. Allowing the wrong thoughts, the wrong ideas, the wrong beliefs (that you refuse to acknowledge or challenge) into your mind can have a tremendous impact on the function of the human body. So you see that the Law of Sanitation also means cleaning the mind. Staying open-minded, and constantly trying to learn, observe, and evolve through our understanding can have a profound impact on our overall health and well-being.

It has been stated that humanity suffers from more than 10,000 known diseases, and yet the remainder of the animal kingdom combined has less than a few hundred. How is this even possible? How can one species in the animal kingdom be plagued by thousands upon thousands of more diseases than all the other animals combined? Maybe this attributes itself to the Law of Sanitation and its impact on letting the wrong ideas, the wrong thoughts, and the wrong concepts into our mind.

You may remember when I discussed earlier the emotional side of the stress triangle. I noted how that side started inside the body and expressed its dysfunction through your anatomy and your body functions. It is fairly easy to see that the other animals in the animal kingdom don't think like we do. They do not reason like we do. You will never see a giraffe write a book or a zebra compose a symphony or even a monkey building a skyscraper. These powers of intellect and reasoning are not gifts that the rest of the animal kingdom enjoys. Only human beings have these special gifts of logic and understanding.

Like all gifts, however, they do need to be understood so that they may be properly utilized to our advantage. If used improperly they can cause as much harm as good. Dr. Fleet, my grandfather, Dr. Zhu, Dr. Frank, and so many more of my mentors all stated that thoughts become things, that your thoughts will become your diseases of tomorrow if not properly dealt with. An adage in healing is that 80 percent or more of all the 10,000 diseases known to man begin within. We lay the groundwork for our very trials and tribulations that we are to undergo. All too often we are responsible for our very own health issues.

A classic case in point to represent this is to look at any number of health issues that have no known cause, or as medicine likes to refer to them, "etiology unknown." Quite often they get lumped under the term "autoimmune disorders," which I tease in practice is a fancy way of saying "I just don't know." If we applied our stress triangle to this idea of disease, what are the odds of all the autoimmune disorders coming from some kind of mechanical trauma? I would think with all the technology that we have today, tests in the hospitals, and the physicians constantly searching, that a mechanical cause of disease would be quite obvious. And what about the chemical or the nutritional side of the triangle? If the cause of your diseases were located there, surely blood panels, urine tests, X-rays, CAT scans, MRIs (and the list goes on and on and on) would be able to find the majority of those problems. Yet this is not the case. It is fully accepted and acknowledged that 80 percent or more of all the diseases that affect mankind begin somewhere outside the mechanical causes or the chemical/nutritional causes. Well, that only leaves one side of that triangle left.

They must be of an emotional suggestive nature which is interfering with normal body function. This means that 80 percent or more of what goes wrong with us is of an energetic, emotional nature. This can prove to be challenging in practice because unlike mechanical and nutritional stress, how do you measure someones thoughts, habits, or acts? Maybe this is why our current health care system often fails so many of its recipients. Modern medicine was invented on a battlefield and is designed to handle acute traumatic injury and infectious diseases. It is very good at that. However, if your condition is not acute, traumatic, or infectious, then our current health care system is often flying blind with its hands tied behind its back, and all it can do is manage the symptoms until eventually the condition consumes its host. I do not accept this. It is one of the primary reasons I got into health care and healing. I thought there had to be another way. And there is.

Healing takes effort. If you want to be well you have to do the things that other well people do. The author Brian Tracy once pointed out that if you wanted to be successful at something all you had to do was follow the exact steps that a successful person has taken. This model has been repeated time and time again with great success. To assume that this would not apply to health and healing seems a bit foolish to me.

If I wanted to lose weight, for example, I would only need to look at someone who is healthy, lean, and fit and copy their routine. If I wanted a more flexible body, I would only need to look at someone who was active and stretched and maintained their flexibility through exercise and movement. If I followed their routine exactly it would only make sense that I would receive similar benefits. If I chose to invest money the way Warren Buffett did and in the same manner that he chose then it would make sense that I also would receive the same benefits. This is where the rubber meets the road.

If you are reading this book and you are sitting there feeling ill, tired, sick, and behind the proverbial eight ball of life, ask yourself if you are willing to do what is necessary to become well. I pointed out in the first part of this chapter that stress is the cause of all disease and dysfunction. I noted that stress comes in three very distinct flavors, the first being a mechanical side that requires physical treatment through movement and manipulation of the body. There are numerous fields in healing that deal with this side alone—orthopedic doctors, physical therapists, chiropractors, massage therapists, bone setters, and the list goes on and on. I then mentioned the nutritional side that tends to be more chemical in nature. Once again there are many, many entry points into healing that specialize in this field. All of pharmacy, all your herbalists, anyone selling a vitamin A mineral or a supplement of any kind, dietitians … they all work on this aspect of the healing triangle.

Then, however, comes the emotional side. This side also has many potential healers involved—psychiatrists, psychologists, psychiatric therapists, psychoanalysis experts, hypnotherapists, ministers, faith healers, counselors, most good physicians, and, once again, the list goes on and on. Where my approach differs from all those listed above is that I choose to look at all three sides of the healing triangle. I pushed myself through my education and my learning and my understanding not to treat one side only but to look at the big picture and see it all. I found time and time again that it was never just one side causing someone's disease or dysfunction. Quite often it was a blend of two or more of the sides of the triangle. Many times the cause would be in one aspect of the healing triangle while its effects would be expressed in another aspect. It's often too easy to get caught up in treating the effect—the symptoms—but never going after the root cause.

I pointed out in practice years ago to some physicians that I was training that we are always treating two patients on every visit. One patient has a cause of a condition that you're searching for and the other patient has effects that are expressing for which they need help to get relief. You're always treating both. By doing this you allow the patient the greatest amount of relief possible, and you're removing the very reason why the symptoms began in the first place. As a healer, this is a game changer. It's how you truly help the body to recover and allow someone to get their life back. This was a primary driving force behind me writing this book.

## THE TEA PRINCIPLE

Several years back I came across this idea of the TEA principle. It was shared with me by one of the gentlemen who learned under Dr. Fleet. He noted that when you need to see something clearly you should take time for TEA. At first, this seemed silly to me. What did he mean? But, upon further investigation, the profoundness of this simple statement really set in with me. It starts with the idea that thoughts become things.

As I mentioned before, get angry and see what your blood pressure does. Or maybe notice the tummy troubles you have when you get worried. If your thoughts physically manifest in your body in the form of symptoms, then you must learn to control your thoughts. The TEA principle is one of the better ways I've found to do this.

It starts by looking at each letter in the word "TEA." T stands for *transmutation*. That word alone can seem confusing, but the simplest definition merely means to transform. It follows one of the first laws of physics that energy can neither be created nor destroyed; it can only be changed. So the first letter in the TEA principle stands for the ability to change something.

When confronted with a stressor, all you need to do is take a moment and asked yourself if you can change this situation. Is it within your power to change it? If you're struggling to go to bed at night, change your routine and turn in earlier. If it is cold and rainy outside, this is beyond your control; you cannot change the weather. Some situations we can change, and if we do so immediately, the problem will cease to exist. However, we often find ourselves faced with a dilemma that is beyond our control.

A problem that we cannot change leads us to the second letter, E, in the TEA principle. The E stands for *elimination*. Is it possible for you to completely eliminate the problem in front of you? If you have a job you don't like, you can quit. If you have a friend that is not so good to you, you can let them go. If you have an old car that's always breaking down, you can get rid of it. The key to the E portion of the TEA principle is to let it go.

Can you let go of the stresses, the emotions, and the problems you face? If you can, do so immediately. Holding onto them overwhelms the system and eventually leads to dysfunction as you suppress all that emotional energy. There are, however, times when we cannot eliminate something, when there's an ill child in the family, for example. In some situations, you cannot change or eliminate their illness, which brings us to A, the final letter in the TEA principle.

The A stands for the ability to adapt. If you are not able to transmute (or change) your problem and it is beyond your control to eliminate your problem (or let it go), then your body will automatically and innately force you to adapt. However, there is a catch. Adaptation expresses in two varieties, either through instinct or through the gift of reason.

Our instincts always express themselves innately. We do not even have to think about them and our negative emotions express under times or duress and great stress. They are hard wired into us for survival and are a part of our DNA. Emotionally our insticts express through anger, worry, fear, frustration, guilt, etc. They tend to be of a low vibrational frequency that has a negative effect on the body and its tissues. Dr. Fleet often referred to these as the laws of the human mind. If you have a negative, thought, then you must also have a positive one. The positives are expressed through reason and quite often are of a much higher vibrational frequency. They are found in our love, our caring, our sympathy for one another, our faith, our hope, our courage. They quite often need to be learned and acquired through experience. Fleet often referred to these as laws of the soul or the psyche.

So here you have two opposing forces. One expresses through instinct and is often very short and rash in its call to action. I liken this in practice to sitting on the front porch with the dog in the middle of spring. Someone goes jogging by and the dog quickly charges the gate, barking as it runs across the lawn. It instinctually expressed its emotions.

The second of the opposing forces expresses itself using the gift of reason, which must be learned and acquired. We do not innately inherit this polished skill. It must be developed through effort and understanding. It would be the equivalent of that same dog watching the jogger run by and, as it began to move, the owner told it to sit. The dog respectfully sat right back down quietly at the owner's side.

The secret to the adaptation portion of the TEA principle is that you get to choose which of these forces you allow the body to express. You get to choose if you want to be angry or if you want to be more patient. You get to choose if you want to be worried or if you want to be more hopeful and understanding. Either way, it's your choice.

The challenge with writing a book like this is trying to keep up with the ever-evolving changes occurring in the health care field. Since I started this adventure in 2019, a lot has happened. Four years ago no one would have ever thought about a pandemic sweeping across the planet and paralyzing our defunct health care system, but that is exactly what has happened.

The SARS-CoV-2 pandemic has brought to light all the things I described in the previous five chapters. It has validated the reason why

I chose to go into the fields of natural healing. For all the wonders that can be found in the medical community, everything from surgeries to medications and emergency care, this field was all but brought to its knees during the pandemic. In one of my favorite movies, *A Knight's Tale*, Count Adhemar tells William Thatcher, "You have been weighed; you have been measured; and you have been found wanting." With the cracks in the system now being brought into the brightness of daylight, we can see clearly where change is needed. We can see how early intervention in health care can serve our population very well, where waiting too long can have catastrophic effects as we end up doing nothing but triage care and managing chronic conditions that eventually take the lives of our family, friends, and loved ones.

When I started this book I really wasn't sure where to go with it. I wanted to open the eyes of the world to let them know that there are many, many health options out there, and you yourself can be one of your options. So as I come to this final chapter, I have decided to help everyone take back their own health, take back their own care. Therefore, I'm going to walk you through one of the single most important tests I feel an individual can run to assess exactly where your body is in real time. But first we have to look into a field called epigenetics.

## EPIGENETICS

Have you ever heard the term *epigenetics* before? Does it mean anything to you? It means a great deal to me as it is served as the crux of my care for more than two decades. When I started into practice nobody even knew what the word meant, but shortly thereafter it became used more and more frequently in scientific and medical circles. Everyone was excited about DNA and the genes. Surely they were responsible for all the unknown diseases and dysfunctions of the human body.

As the genome study finished up around 2007, the medical community assumed that they would find the answers to all the diseases that had evaded our detection for so many years. This, however, was not to be the case. What they ended up discovering was that human beings have roughly 25,000 genes—but so do rats and monkeys. As a matter of fact, we all share almost exactly the same 25,000 genes. Then why do we look different than a rat?

What was discovered after the genome study was completed was that each gene had the ability to express itself in more than 2,000 unique and different ways. I often liken this to a room full of children who are all given the same 2,000 Lego bricks. When the children are done playing and building all the wonderful things that they can create, we see that no child has built the exact same thing as any other child. All their designs are unique and special. This is exactly how DNA works. Now we must ask ourselves how it's possible that we even have humans then. There must be something more. Enter the field of epigenetics.

What we learned with the genome study and the study of DNA is that DNA has no real true ability to express or activate itself. It is really nothing more than a library book on a shelf loaded with tons of information, but worthless unless someone or something removes it from the shelf, opens it, and begins reading. Epigenetics is the study of the field that begins the reading.

In a nutshell "epigenetics" means "above the gene." It is the study of the signals being received by the receptors on the cell from the environment they're forced to live in. We know now that the surface of the cell has upwards of 150,000 unique receptors. Each time some signal from the environment comes into one of those receptors, the cell responds. Imagine it affecting 10, 15, 1,000, or 10,000 receptors at once. Think of all the possibilities that could occur. The combinations are endless. There's a catch, however.

We have learned that the signals affecting the receptors of the cell only come in three varieties: by way of a mechanical force or trauma, by way of a chemical signal (or are blocked by way of a chemical signal), and as a form of pure energy in a vibrational format. Sound familiar? I often tease in practice that MEN are the cause of all STRESS, and STRESS is the CAUSE of all DISEASE and DYSFUNCTION. Mechanical energy, emotional energy, and nutritional or chemical energy are the only things that can possibly affect the cell receptors and thus allow the DNA to express itself in response to its environment. What if you could tell how the body is attempting to adapt to the environment you're forcing it to live in? After all, the body is roughly 50 trillion cells.

I've spent my career searching for answers, searching for the truth that I knew was out there. It has proven elusive at times, but as I entered into this new decade, the truth began to shine through. And it came in the form of an integrated urinalysis panel (IUP).

By the mid-2010s, I had been teaching digestive work and nutrition to physicians for the better part of 15 years under the tutelage of Dr. Howard Loomis. I often ran across physicians who were desperately seeking answers to help their patients with chronic diseases like diabetes, autoimmune disorders, and GI problems. These physicians had grown weary of the wait-and-see model, and the medicate-and-manage system that they had become accustomed to. They were tired of watching patient after patient succumb to the very diseases that they had been treating.

I watched as functional medicine clinics started springing up across the country. Physicians from all disciplines were flocking to a more natural way to assist their patients. However, the same old methodology was still in place. The "take this for that" model was the dominant method of thinking used by the semi "new" field of functional medicine doctors. They had literally gone from using blood work to assess pathology, to using blood work to look at hormones and vitamin deficiencies and imbalances. Salivary panels and hair analysis became the darlings of the functional medicine field as a generation of doctors scrambled to help their patients with bioidentical hormones, vitamins, minerals, and just about anything else. However, as this field would quickly see, the "take this for that" model really didn't work any better using quasi-natural products instead of pharmaceuticals. Something was still missing.

Part of the problem starts here: Hormones and vitamins are still not true nutrition. You cannot pick vitamin C off a tree anywhere in nature.

You cannot walk up to a bush and pull a little vitamin E off it. You cannot milk vitamin B from a cow. Therefore, all these products have to be obtained through a supplement form, and therein lies the problem. Supplementing nutrition means just that. You can only supplement the diet, not replace it. This fact often appears to be forgotten in the world of healing. All the new blood work and hormone panels were merely damage assessments. They did not serve as an early warning siren telling the body to run and hide or to get out of the way of the truck barreling down the road. They worked to tell you what was already broken.

Now imagine you could tell beforehand that trouble was coming. What if you could be notified to get out of the road before the truck ever gets to you? This is exactly what the IUP does. It is an **epigenetic profile** test that uses two unique panels which notify the individual and their physician of where the body is being pushed too hard and struggling to maintain health, and how the body is trying to respond to the signals from the environment it is being forced to live in.

The IUP is hands down the single greatest test any person could run to truly know how their body is trying to survive and where it might already be broken. The IUP is not merely a damage assessment. It serves as both the Ghost of Christmas Past, by showing you things that are broken and damaged, and as the Ghost of Christmas Future, by guiding you to where and how the body is trying to defend itself from the stresses of its life choices before the damage is done.

## WHAT IS AN IUP?

The Integrated Urinalysis Panel (IUP) consists of 24 tests and assessments placed into two very specific panels. The first half of the tests look for pathologies and imbalances. You read it in the same manner that you would blood work. Think of it as a yellow blood test; it tells us as much as bloodwork, however, instead of blood telling the story, we let urine do so. It is looking for anything that may already be broken. Pathology always trumps anything else that needs to be addressed in one's care. First and foremost, you have to fix the obvious things affecting your health.

If, for example, ketones or glucose are showing up in the pathology portion of the exam, then those things should be addressed immediately by looking for a potential cause. If you ignore these things, they can sink the boat before you can patch the hole. It does little good to pump air into a tire that has a hole the size of a baseball in it. Once pathology has been addressed, then you can look into the real meat and potatoes of the exam.

The second half of the test is assessing digestion. This panel looks at how food enters into the system, moves throughout it, gets utilized, and then removed. In a nutshell, you are analyzing if the body can digest and absorb its nutrients and then eliminate its waste. You are looking at what the body is holding onto and what it is throwing away. Can the body actually use the fuel you are giving it and remove the exhaust it produces? The IUP is the only real-time test that I know of that can assess how the body is trying to maintain homeostasis in the environment and world you're forcing it to live in.

With that basic explanation of why the IUP is important, let's dig a little deeper into the tests themselves. Let's pop the hood and take a look at the IUP engine. As you recall, we noted that the IUP consists of two panels. One deals primarily with pathology and the second deals in early warning signals for trouble that may be brewing ahead.

The first panel, or the "**Ghost of Christmas Past**," is very standard and well known throughout the medical communities. It begins by looking at height, weight, age, and standard medical information. It then assesses the color of the urine, as well as its turbidity. Color can indicate numerous problems trying to express throughout the body. Everything from medications, to bacterial infections, red blood cells, certain types of anemia, and liver dysfunction can all be observed in the color aspect of the IUP.

The turbidity, which is really just a fancy word for "cloudiness," can pick up fat, epithelial cells, blood, pus, and numerous other compounds stressing the system. Things such as glucose, protein, bilirubin, nitrites, ketones, blood, urobilinogen, and leukocytes are all examined as well. If the body is under duress and the kidneys or biliary system are being taxed, then this portion of the panel will often send up a red flag. Dietary stresses like ketosis or even infection can often present in this portion of the IUP. These things can prove invaluable to the physician as they are attempting to assist the patient in regaining their health.

With this said, the lion's share of the patients who walk through my door seldom have pathologies inhibiting their health. The majority of them are suffering from subclinical problems which elude the pathological exams. To put it in another way, they walk into the doctor's office and tell the doctor all the myriad of symptoms that they are suffering from. The doctor then runs numerous tests on them only to find nothing is broken. The patient is then sent home with or without some form of prescription and instructed to "wait and see." How often have we all been part of this? It is not your physician's fault because the model they are trained in is a triage -based system. It's wonderful at traumas, accidents, and infectious disease, but if that's not your problem, then you're barking up the wrong tree.

This brings us to the second panel of the IUP, the "**Ghost of Christmas Future**"!

This is where the true magic of the IUP shows itself. Each test reads like a unique musical note. When strung together, the notes play a song that is very specific and individualized to the person being tested. No two songs are exactly the same. Every individual arrived at their dysfunctions in their own special way. The IUP serves as a road map to exactly how the body is attempting to resist the stresses feeding into the patient's dysfunction. By definition, this is exactly what epigenetics and epigenetic testing is meant to represent: a real time look into how the body is functioning and adapting to the environment that it is forced to exist in.

Now let us take a closer look at the individual tests making up the second panel of the IUP. The first test is looking at something known as **indicanuria**, a collection of 38 different chemicals produced in the

GI tract by both proper and improper food breakdown and opportunistic critters such as yeast and bacteria. These byproduct chemicals are considered toxic and poisonous to the human body. Quite often, in an attempt to rid itself of these toxins, the body will draw them back inside into circulation and filter them out through the kidneys and urine. If this process gets overwhelmed, it can lead to a bowel toxicity. Symptoms can range from fatigue to bloating, gas, and bowel unrest (as in loose stools or constipation). Malabsorption syndromes, putrefaction, biliary obstruction, and numerous other conditions involving the skin, moods, fatigue, and toxicity can often be found when the indicanuria levels are outside normal range. In advanced cases, autoimmune disorders often are paired with this test, along with popular terms like "leaky gut syndrome" and the numerous symptoms associated with that. Clinically, if the indicanuria is allowed to persist for too long, you will often see a weakening in the abdominal musculature and a rounded or protruding abdomen. A quick pat of the tummy or a side profile view in the bathroom mirror might give you a hint.

The next test on the sheet is known as **total sediment**. It is a look into how the body is burning and utilizing the food choices you give it. It focuses on the macro nutrients such as carbohydrates, fats, and proteins and how the body burns each of those fuels for energy and produces a waste product. If those fuels are burned cleanly, then the body is quite happy. However, if the digestive mechanism is out of rhythm and running too fast or too slow then the fuels it is attempting to use are burned inefficiently and dirty.

Imagine a small vehicle like a Prius getting 50 miles to the gallon and burning clean. This is what we're trying to achieve, but when dysfunction sets in, we often find ourselves sitting behind a city bus spewing out black smoke and exhaust into the environment as it leaves the stoplight. Where does all that exhaust and pollution go? How does it get outside the body? Or does it simply just go a little further inside, causing more and more disruption of a healthy system?

As we leave total sediment, we are brought to the next test, which is titled **calcium**. This test often—and mistakenly—looks at calcium only, which could not be more wrong. It is looking at mineralization of the body. Does your body have an adequate supply of all the minerals it needs to function properly? If not, why not? This is a wonderful test because it is not just looking at minerals but rather at circulation. You will often see toxicity, glandular disturbances, blood pressure problems, cholesterol imbalances, hormonal disruptions, vitamin and mineral deficiencies, and stiff, sore, and achy joints showing up when this particular music note goes flat.

This brings us to the **pH** test, a greatly misunderstood section of laboratory science. So many people are trying to alkalize their pH. Time and again you hear of one person or another saying, "If I'm too acidic I'll get cancer, and I need to change that." This statement can be very misleading as the body has 10 times the acid-producing functions as it does alkaline-producing functions. Therefore, it makes sense that the urine might want to be somewhat acidic in order to assist the blood in maintaining its alkaline properties. Let us look at this in a different way.

The pH can be confusing, so, for simplicity, let's change "acids" and "bases" into "hot" and "cold." Imagine a pH of 7.0 is room temperature. Since we often think of "acids" as being able to burn us, we will refer to them as being "hot." Bases, then, will represent things that are "cold." Anything above 7.0 (for example, a pH of 7.4) would be "cold." Anything below 7.0 we could consider "hot." Once you observe this, it can be understood that the blood must maintain a pH of 7.4, which is slightly alkaline (or cold for our purpose of discussion).

This would be like trying to keep your house at exactly 74 degrees all the time. If it's 100 outside, it still has to stay at 74. Not 75! Not 73! But it must stay at 74! To most of you this would seem an impossibility as the furnace or the air conditioner is always kicking on and off in an attempt to maintain this equilibrium. And yet, this is exactly what the body is designed to do. Its creator knew that it would have to maintain the 7.4 pH of the blood at all times. Otherwise the results would be catastrophic and hospitalization would be sure to follow.

In order to do this, it allowed for the body to change its temperature, its pH of its urine, and its concentration of solutes like salts, electrolytes, and minerals quite rapidly. Basically, it allowed for the body to open the windows on the house and air things out, or shut it up completely to keep that temperature exact. Therefore, the pH of the urine is best set right below room temperature at a slightly acidic level of around 6.6. Dysfunction in this particular test always shows in the digestive system. If the pH is off, either high or low, you can bet digestive disturbance will not be far behind.

This brings us to the **chloride** test. Many of you have heard of sodium chloride in table salt, and this is really not that different. It's looking at electrolyte imbalances throughout the body. It's focusing on the adrenal gland and how it's responding to the stresses and the signals coming in from the environment. Of course, it'll also pick up stress on proper kidney function and water reabsorption. Chronic fatigue, sleeplessness, irritability, restlessness, forgetfulness, malaise, and lethargy can all rear their little ugly heads under this one test.

From the chloride test we are led to the **volume** test, which measures the amount of urine excreted over 24 hours. As a diagnostic test, urine has been studied for centuries. (Human beings have really not changed that much.) One Canadian study found that the average sample of urine contains more than 3,000 chemicals in its makeup. However, most medical testing fails to look at anything beyond a simple chem strip test.

The IUP excels at looking into the integration and removal of food and waste particles from the body. Due to the stability and the consistency of our urine, it serves as a wonderful test. The volume average thus acts as a great barometer for health, and because the urine is quite stable, sterile, and well documented in the medical literature, the amount excreted over a 24-hour period is easily measured and very reliable.

With this in mind, a set, measurable amount of urine is to be released every 24 hours. If the volume falls outside this range, either high or low, then through questioning and an examination it can be determined if some type of dysfunction is occurring and why. For example, an excessively high urine volume, termed as polyuria, could be due to excessive fluid intake such as sugar-free drinks, colas, alcohol, coffees, teas, water etc. Diuretics and numerous other medications can also increase urinary output. On the flip side, a decrease in volume can indicate dehydration, poor kidney function, or other pathologies. Whether it is high or low, the body is demonstrating an attempt to push back against a stress in its environment. It does not care if that stress is self-induced (like dehydration) or if it's a poison or toxin (like a drug). Either way, knowledge is gained and the patient is the better for it.

**Specific gravity** is the next test to be run in the panel, and it looks at the ability of the kidneys to concentrate the waste in the urine. Quite often in practice I describe this test in relation to the volume. The volume often indicates the amount of water you put in a mopping bucket to clean your floors. The specific gravity is looking at how dirty the water became once you finished mopping. The volume and the specific gravity are inversely proportional. Meaning they are like two ends of a teeter-totter. As one goes down the other should go up, and vice versa. Problems arise when this does not occur. Much can be gleaned by looking at specific gravity and its relationship to volume. Poor kidney function, chronic sensitivity to smoke, perfumes, and smells, allergies, low back pain, swelling and edema, and lymphatic function are just a few of the things you look for when these two tests are out of harmony with one another.

We are now coming to the last three tests in the panel. By now it is fairly easy to see how much can be learned about a body and its overall health with a simple IUP. Imagine being able to see where the body is getting itself into trouble before the trouble actually begins. How invaluable would this knowledge be?

We now come to the **color change** test, one of the more unique tests of the panel. Clinical experience over the years has taught us quite a bit about its importance. As humanity has evolved in its dietary choices and use of medications, the color change test has become more and more important.

When a reagent is added to the urine sample, the colors can range from no change to a rainbow of choices, from reds to purples to white, etc. Each change indicates a different stress challenging the GI tract. Painkillers, antacids, antibiotics, and microbiome disruptions, along with numerous other toxins, can all demonstrate their effects on the health of the body and its GI tract. It is not uncommon to see the effects of yeast overgrowth with this particular test. Fatigue, lethargy, skin irritations, mood swings, brain fog or forgetfulness, and intense cravings for sweets often show up when the color change is outside normal range.

The **vitamin C** test. It was not long ago that Dr. Loomis, one of my mentors, gave a talk on the side effects presented with scurvy. The old British naval journals were full of stories describing the horrific side effects that plagued much of the sailing world in the late 16th century. An unnamed English ship surgeon wrote of his experience with this disease:

> "It rotted all my gums, which gave out a black and putrid blood. My thighs and lower legs were black and gangrenous, and I was forced to use my knife each day to cut into the flesh in order to release this black and foul blood. I also use my knife on my gums, which were livid and growing over my teeth. When I had cut away this dead flesh and caused much black blood to flow, I rinsed my mouth and teeth with my urine rubbing them very hard. And the unfortunate thing was that I could not eat, desiring more to swallow than to chew. Many of our people died of it every day, and we saw bodies thrown into the sea constantly, three or four at a time."

Fortunately, we no longer live in the 16th century and vitamin C is now plentiful throughout the world and in our diet. After all, we fortify everything with vitamins and minerals. But what if you couldn't digest it? What if you ate plenty of foods rich in vitamin C but your body had an issue with breaking it down and absorbing it? This would bring us back to Dr. Loomis' discussion.

He noted the symptoms of a vitamin C deficiency. We can all quickly recall the bleeding gums, but those tend to come on much later as the disease advances. The bedridden effects and death all present in the late stages of the disease. What Dr. Loomis did that was so outstanding was to describe the early symptoms of vitamin C deficiency: fatigue; stiff, sore, achy joints and muscles; sinus irritation; circulation problems; and visual disturbances, along with the immune weakness which often preceded the bleeding gums, the tissue rotting, and the eventual death mentioned by the ship's surgeon.

Now fast forward to today. Vitamin C is a five-carbon sugar in its chemical makeup. Because it's a sugar, it is therefore considered a carbohydrate. Imagine someone having trouble absorbing or utilizing carbohydrates in their diet. It would be safe to theorize that they might have trouble utilizing a carbohydrate vitamin. Since vitamin C is so abundant in our diet, we would seldom see full-blown scurvy in its advanced stages. However, I think it is safe to theorize that it might present itself in its earlier forms.

Theoretically, it might look something like this: Someone could have a stiff, sore, achy back with no trauma or maybe chronic sinusitis coupled with chronic fatigue. They would always be catching colds or somewhat under the weather, and they might even have a blood pressure problem. Heck, throw in some seasonal allergies and a skin irritation like eczema, and you would likely have a vitamin C disruption in the body. All you would need now is to brush and floss your teeth and notice a little blood when you rinse your mouth. But I digress. It's just a theory.

We have now arrived at the **non-protein nitrogen** test, the final one in the IUP panel, which is a catabolic index test. Basically, it asks whether the body is in an anabolic state, where it is building tissue rapidly, or in a metabolic state, where it's trying to maintain itself. Anabolic states can be desirable in young children who are growing rapidly or in women who are pregnant.

The catabolic state is never desired. It indicates that the body is tearing down itself in an effort to get fuel for energy to survive. You will see this in degenerative diseases like cancers and tuberculosis. The effects of catabolism on the body are far-reaching. It can affect blood pH in an alkaline direction. It can cause the digestive tract to express a loose stool (interfering with the utilization of nutrients), insomnia, lymphatic congestion, increased aging, and connective tissue breakdown.

The metabolic state is one in which the body is maintaining itself against the world we are forcing it to live in. This is the most desired state and the one we often try to achieve. As you can see, the non-protein nitrogen test can serve as a wonderful indicator of current body health.

Now that we have had a chance to look at the components of the IUP, let us take it out for a test drive in a real world scenario with real people and real patients.

Randy came into my office for a first time visit. He wasn't really sure what to expect as he had been referred there by several of his friends, but he had really never heard of me. We sat during our first consultation and I began to take my notes. I follow a technique called mind mapping, which I am quite fond of. It allows me to take a history of the patient in a concise manner. At any point on future visits, I can glance at my mind map and get a thorough reminder of exactly why the patient is here and the problems they are facing. I begin my notes in the center of a page by writing ***perfect health.*** After all, this is what everyone is truly after. If you have perfect health there can be nothing wrong with you. It therefore serves as a wonderful centerpiece for what that patient is trying to achieve and accomplish.

On Randy's visit, I could see that he was clearly uncomfortable as he seemed unsettled and as if he was in pain. I began by asking, "What brought you in today?" He started listing the health issues which troubled him the most as I feverishly took my notes. He began by noting that he had suffered from intense bladder pain and urinary frequency for more than a decade. The pain would shoot and stab across his pelvis every time he had to urinate or even felt that he might have to. Randy had been to multiple specialists and urologists in an effort to find some answers. Numerous medications, scopes, and pain relievers found him in the same position he was in when he started on his journey.

He went on to mention that he was also suffering from severe anxiety, lifelong sinus problems, chronic low back pain and a skyrocketing blood pressure that his doctors just could not seem to get under control. After a short conversation, I assured Randy that he had come to the right place. I recommended running a series of tests in my office, and I immediately referred him to an IUP. Here are those results.

Randy's pathology section of the IUP panel was relatively unremarkable. Before me sat a man who had suffered for a decade from unrelenting pelvic pain and urinary irritation, and yet the portion of lab work that shows what's broken was relatively clean. There was a trace amount of protein and a trace amount of blood. Both of which would indicate an irritation and a stress on the urinary tract, the kidneys, or the bladder. But it was only a trace and not usually a huge problem. The only other thing that showed up in the pathology were leukocytes (white blood cells). As I mentioned earlier in the chapter, those white blood cells can indicate infection or a chronic irritation in the body caused by some inflammatory process. Infection had been ruled out by his other physicians so I knew I was looking at unchecked inflammation within the body.

Here's where things started to get interesting. The second panel on the IUP served to be incredibly eye opening. The **indican** levels were outside normal range and elevated. I immediately knew I had a patient who was having trouble with an elimination issue, but according to the IUP it looked as though toxicity might be occurring not only in the urinary tract but in the GI tract as well. Thoughts started going through my head. Could his whole body possibly be toxic and inflamed? I proceeded on.

Next I looked at the **total sediment** test, which was also elevated. The calcium oxalate levels were three times higher than normal, and experience had taught me to start looking for the possibility of kidney stone formation, biliary dysfunction, or some other chronic irritation in the urinary tract. As I proceeded further into the IUP, I noticed the calcium levels were below normal, indicating poor circulation of both nutrients and waste removal. I started thinking, *I've got a patient who's not utilizing his diet properly, struggling to break that diet down once it gets inside the body, and having a challenge delivering the nutrients to the cells and removing their waste.* It was a classic case of bowel toxicity or what is often referred to in medical literature as leaky gut syndrome. I proceeded on.

The next several tests were unremarkable and within normal limits until we arrived at the **chloride** test. The chloride levels were lower than normal, indicating the possibility of stress on the adrenal glands. You may remember that the adrenal glands help the body to regulate a hormone known as cortisol, which allows you to control anxiety and mood swings. Things were starting to line up, and I knew we were on the right track.

The **volume** test followed next and was above normal but not excessively. Where things became more interesting was when I compared the volume test to the **specific gravity**. As you may recall, the specific gravity test measures how the kidneys are able to concentrate the urine and remove waste from inside the body. In Randy's case the gravity was almost nonexistent, which meant the kidneys were just not doing their job. All the toxicity produced by the body was remaining inside and desperately searching for another way out. The indicanuria test had already let me know that the bowels were not keeping up with waste removal on that end of things, and now here we sat with the kidneys on the other end also not doing their job. Over two decades of practice has clinically taught me that when the bowels and the urine cannot handle waste removal, the **lungs**, **skin**, and **sinuses** will try to do it for you. What I failed to mention above was that Randy also noted a lifelong battle with chronic sinus irritation, folliculitis on his scalp, and a small recurring cough for more than 20 years that just never seemed to go away. At this point I was quite excited. I often tell my patients if it walks like a duck, quacks like a duck, and you see feathers, odds are pretty good you might have a duck! And it was sure looking like I had one here.

The **color change** test was relatively unremarkable, while the **vitamin C** test was slightly elevated. As you may recall in our description of the vitamin C test, it is a fuel for the adrenal glands which aids the body in handling stress and controlling anxiety and mood swings. The last test involving the **non-protein nitrogen** Test was within normal limits.

I sat with Randy and went over his results just like I did here with you, my reader. When we finished I told him that I believed I had found the cause of his effects and I understood why other physicians before me had not seen it. They were looking only where their training could take them, for what was broken but not at how the body was trying to adapt.

Shortly after this, we began care. I am proud to say that after a decade of bladder problems and pelvic pain, Randy is pain free! His urinary tract is functioning normally and no longer an issue. His moods have changed for the better. His blood pressure is now running 120/78, perfectly normal. He has seen no return of the folliculitis on the scalp, and all those pestering chronic sinus infections and coughs have moved on. At time of writing, it has been more than three years since Randy first came to me. His life has totally changed, and today he is medication free. I end every one of my radio show episodes with this statement, "If you don't expect a miracle they tend not to happen." Randy had the faith and belief that he could be better. He expected his miracle, and it absolutely happened!

There you have it. This concludes my brief description of the IUP and how and why it works so well. Each individual test holds a significant importance in its own right and should be appreciated. However, the real art comes in when a skillful clinician can string together the tests, note by note, into a song, seeing how each individual panel can lead into the next and present the true functioning of the body. This is a skill set that only a few clinicians have. I have built my entire career around this ability to understand and interpret what the body is trying to say. If one can listen, one can truly learn. And this is where true healing can be found.

Hopefully you can now see why this test is so very important. As I mentioned above, epigenetics is the study of how your actions and choices affect the expression of your genes and your DNA. In today's world, where we are constantly discussing genetic flaws and genetic tendencies, I cannot imagine a more important test to demonstrate how and where your body is pushing back against the stresses of your environment. Imagine how fantastic it would be if you could intervene early in your body's expression before it progressed into a disease state. Think of all the heartaches and sorrow that come from the diagnosis of conditions that could have been prevented had you just known.

Penn State University completed a very interesting study on chronic degenerative diseases. They found that more than 80 percent of all the diseases that plague mankind could be avoided through lifestyle adaptations, dietary change, and the right thinking. Look around at all of your loved ones who have suffered needlessly over the years, chasing this symptom or that, only to become more and more miserable as their health—and their finances—dwindled away. I started writing this book in an effort to help people to regain their lives, to help people overcome all the obstacles and trials put before them. I truly felt all they needed was a little more knowledge and, with that in hand, they could reclaim the person they once were. The IUP serves as my base in understanding how the body is responding to all the stresses in someone's life.

# CONCLUSION

Throughout my 25 years hosting a radio show, and through my social media channels, I've found that most folks want to know where they can get my kind of care. Is there a doctor I can refer them to? The issue is that there isn't a practitioner in the world that practices just like me. This isn't my ego speaking. After my traditional doctorate, I've spent the last 25 years studying with some of the brightest minds in the healing arts, in some of the most remote locations, with intense dedication. I didn't go through just one institution to get this education. I pieced it together from dozens of them. In my first few years of practice, I found that not one system I had studied was complete; they all had holes. However, they all had some amazing benefits! I took the best parts of those systems, and weaved them together with other systems, while also creating my own proprietary systems and adding those into my care. Therefore, it is very difficult for a physician to replicate my education, unless I teach them. It's taken me 25 years. Someday I hope to teach, but for now, patients come first. My time is spent in practice. Any little time I have left continues my education, promotes and increases my media presence and message, and is spent with my wife and son.

So what can you do? You've read the book, you understand my message, what's next? Well, the easiest and most practical solution would be to find a physician that can help you with your emotional health, nutritional health, and your mechanical health. That would be your best bet. However, this would constitute having three different providers, no doubt with conflicting opinions sometimes, so it may be a bit of a challenge. I provide care for all three sides of the MEN triangle I've mentioned. Most don't.

The one piece of my care I can easily share, without a patient being in front of me, is the integrated urinalysis panel (IUP). It is (and always has been) an at-home laboratory test. For 25 years, I have owned and operated the only integrated urinalysis laboratory in the world. I have shipped urinalysis kits to physicians for their own patients; and, of course, I offer it in my own care, to my own patients.

When a patient first comes to see me, they have a consultation. Then, if they decide they like what they hear and want to move forward, I do a series of tests, called a workup. The workup is a series of three tests, two of which have to be run manually in office, but the third, the IUP, does not. And as you can see, there is a tremendous amount of valuable information in this laboratory test. From the workup, I do a report of findings or a second consultation going over the results from the workup. Then they decide if they want to move forward with care. If they do, they start seeing me in office once a week, usually for a series of 12 weeks. After care is done, we reevaluate their progress and determine if their condition is resolved or still requires more care. We do an additional 12 weeks of in-person care. In the report of findings, I will be able to tell them how many series of care I think they will need to get at the issues. Big cases will typically require more than 12 weeks of care. That is an in-office care model.

For those patients that do not live locally, I offer a solution called concierge care, which is simply a concentrated form of the workup and care received through weekly office visits. Patients are seen over a three-day period. The appointments are scheduled off hours over a Friday, Saturday, and Sunday, since they are too long to fit into my regular schedule. I condense 12 weeks of care into a three-day period involving several longer appointments.

Currently, I have a waitlist for virtual patients. Virtual care has proved tricky for me to provide, because what I do in office, hands on, in front of a patient, is a valuable piece of the success of my care. There are certain things that are very difficult to do virtually. I'm currently in the process of creating a virtual program, as many people have asked for this, that will enable me to still provide the same level of care that my patients receive in office. For now, I am still working on this and it may be that I have to do a hybrid model, where there are a few visits in person during care while the majority can be done virtually. Once I hone this process and I feel comfortable that it will be successful for every patient, and meet my own expectations of my care, I can roll it out. Until then, I will not bring to market something that I am not yet comfortable with.

That said, I am without a doubt comfortable with the IUP. That model has always been an at-home test; the process and shipping logistics I've already been doing. What I have not done is make it available to purchase for any individual around the country. Typically, it would take a trained physician to interpret the results for you and order your test. Over the last several years, I have worked to create a software system that can interpret the lab in the specific way that I do and create a report that makes sense to the patient—to create their story, to sing their song, in a way that they can understand without me being right in front of them.

As it exists for the physician, the IUP is a collection of data and graphs that would make no sense to the average lay person. When I go over an IUP with patients, I have the ability to analogize, and to interpret their story for them quickly and easily. I have probably interpreted 250,000 IUPs for my own patients, and for the patients of physicians across the country, over the last 25 years. All I needed was a software system that could do that for me, which would grow my reach of care and access to the IUP exponentially.

Today, I am happy to announce, after years in the making, that I have created a new division of our laboratory to do just that! ePeeGen is the name of our at home laboratory testing division, which enters the at-home laboratory testing market to help individuals seeking care who just cannot seem to find the answers they are looking for. At-home lab testing was growing in market share before COVID-19. After COVID-19, the floodgates opened with at-home everything! After watching the cornucopia of tests and cure-all accusations pouring into the market, I felt it was time for a sound and proven laboratory test to be made accessible to the public. My message has remained clear for more than two decades: Help as many people as you possibly can to reclaim their lives so that they can live life to its fullest. And now we are finally ready to be a part of doing just that!

That mission is why we have expanded our work – not just through cutting edge lab testing, but through the development of my own supplement line. Created to support ePeeGen lab testing, my supplement line, ePeeWell, offers natural healing solutions and support. In total, there will be 7 products. Of those 7 products, as I write this, one formulation is complete and it is my gold star, the supplement everyone can benefit from, Elixir-Vitae. Toxins are an unavoidable part of modern life, and our health depends on our ability to detox, repair and rebuild at the cellular level. That's why I formulated Elixir-Vitae, a powerful blend of nature's best detoxifiers and rejuvenators, featuring Pine Pollen, Chlorella, Spirulina, and Milk Thistle – each carefully chosen to support hormonal balance, boost immunity, and promote deep cellular healing.

Now with ePeeGen's advanced home testing and Elixir-Vitae's natural healing power, we are ready to help even more people uncover the root causes of their health challenges and take control of their well-being. This is just the beginning – your journey to vibrant health starts now!

If you are interested in ordering the IUP or Elixir-Vitae, to take the first steps in reclaiming your health go to: http://epeegen.com/.

Thank you for taking the time to read this book, I hope you found it a helpful, eye-opening resource on how to keep your body as healthy as possible!

Remember …

If you don't expect a miracle, they tend not to happen.

## McCaffrey Health Center

3330 Hedley Road
Ste. C
Springfield, IL 62711
217-726-0151

info@mccaffreyhealth.com
https://www.mccaffreyhealth.com/
http://epeegen.com/

Watch Dr. Sean's "House Call" radio show live on our Facebook page every Saturday at 8am CST.

## Follow Dr. Sean on his social channels:

**Facebook** - https://www.facebook.com/McCaffreyHealthCenter
**Instagram** - https://www.instagram.com/drseanmccaffrey/
**YouTube** - https://www.youtube.com/@dr.seanmccaffrey4616

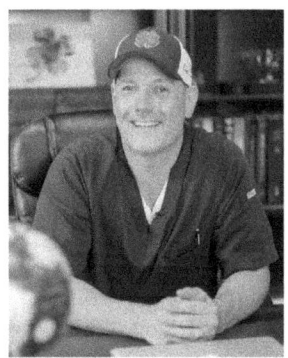

Dr. Sean McCaffrey is a practicing physician of 25 years. He has created a unique style of holistic healthcare to combat chronic and degenerative disease. Our current medical system has failed miserably with chronic disease. 80% of us will pass from it and we have the most expensive healthcare system in the world, that cures nothing, only manages symptoms.

Sean has really become a healing historian, with modern clinical experience. The man is not only a practicing physician, he is a professional student, that has dedicated his life to understanding how the human body acquires disease. In the 25 years since his formal doctorate, he has dedicated himself to the educational equivalent of about 3 more doctorates. These have not been from formal institutions of learning. They have come from 25 years of seeking global healing styles, and old world healers and systems, that our medical model moved away from, or ignored. After studying dozens of them and then clinically testing them, he wove together their common threads and has created something truly remarkable.

As mentioned, 80% of us will pass from something chronic and degenerative. Many suffer daily from debilitating symptoms of chronic disease. Many suffer in silence. This book is the story of the creation of his style of care, and a wealth of information on how our current healthcare model began, how it's going (not well), and what is possible when we step outside of it's matrix. McCaffrey Health Center is the practice name. He is a radio show host of 25 years as well.

www.ingramcontent.com/pod-product-compliance
Lightning Source LLC
Chambersburg PA
CBHW041039050426
42337CB00059B/5077